Preparing for FDA Pre-Approval Inspections

DRUGS AND THE PHARMACEUTICAL SCIENCES

DRUGS AND THE PHARMACEUTICAL SCIENCES

A Series of Textbooks and Monographs

Preparing for FDA Pre-Approval Inspections

edited by

Martin D. Hynes III
Eli Lilly and Company
Indianapolis, Indiana

MARCEL DEKKER, INC.   NEW YORK · BASEL

Library of Congress Cataloging-in-PublicationData

Preparing for FDA pre-approval inspections / edited by Martin D. Hynes, III.
    p.   cm.— (Drugs and the pharmaceutical sciences; v. 93)
    Includes index.
    ISBN 0-8247-0218-2 (alk. paper)
    1. Drugs—Research—Standards—United States. 2. United States. Food and Drug
Administration. I. Hynes, Martin D. II. Series.
RM301.27.P74 1998
615'.19—dc21   98-27750
                                                                   CIP

This book is printed on acid-free paper.

Headquarters
Marcel Dekker, Inc.
270 Madison Avenue, New York, NY 10016
tel: 212-696-9000; fax: 212-685-4540

Eastern Hemisphere Distribution
Marcel Dekker AG
Hutgasse 4, Postfach 812, CH-4001 Basel, Switzerland
tel: 44-61-261-8482; fax: 44-61-261-8896

World Wide Web
http://www.dekker.com

The publisher offers discounts on this book when ordered in bulk quantities. For more information, write to Special Sales/Professional Marketing at the headquarters address above.

Current printing (last digit)
10 9 8 7 6 5

PRINTED IN THE UNITED STATES OF AMERICA

*To my wife Lynn
and my children Amy and Katie
for their love and support*

Preface

During the 1989 generic-drug scandal, the Food and Drug Administration (FDA) discovered that a number of firms had committed fraud in the conduct of bioavailability and bioequivalence studies. It was further found that generic firms had misrepresented study data, facilities, and manufacturing processes. The FDA also concluded that production problems could be traced to inadequate product development. As a result of these findings, the FDA significantly increased its focus on product development activities.

Evidence of this increased focus on the part of the FDA first emerged in the mid-Atlantic region in the form of the 1990 mid-Atlantic Regional Drug Inspection Program authored by Henry Avellon. This regional inspection program led to the development of an FDA-wide pre-approval inspection program that applied to both generic and ethical firms. This program was summarized in the FDA Compliance Program Guidance Manual (7346.832) on Pre-Approval Drug Inspections/Investigations that was officially issued in 1990. This inspection manual for human drugs was revised in 1994. The program was expanded in 1991 to cover animal drugs as well as human drugs.

Introduction of this pre-approval inspection program represented significant change in the approval process for new chemical entities (NCEs) and generic drugs, in that for the first time the field/district compliance branch of the FDA was directly involved in the process of approving drugs for commercial use. Prior to this FDA initiative, only the Center for Drug Evaluation and Research (CDER) reviewed and approved marketing applications. Thus, a new and second hurdle was introduced to the drug approval process. The imposition of this additional hurdle resulted in numerous (and at times lengthy) delays in drug approvals. In the 12-month period ending in March 1991, approval was withheld on 65% of the applications reviewed by the FDA field offices. The rate at which approvals have been withheld has declined over the past several years to approximately 30% in

1997. Although this represents marked improvement over the early years, the rate is still disturbingly high. These delays not only are costly to the firms bringing new drugs to the market but they slow the availability of new therapies to patients in need. It is therefore important to further decrease the rate at which the field offices are recommending delay in approval.

The aim of this book is to help those involved in product development understand FDA requirements for the manufacture of clinical trial material and product development activities. Additionally, it describes what the FDA will look for during the conduct of the inspection.

The book also outlines strategies that various firms have utilized to successfully prepare for pre-approval inspections. These strategies range from activities that can take place in the weeks and months prior to an inspection to longer-term approaches to product development during the years prior to an inspection. The goal of these strategies is to minimize delays in approval.

I am indebted to my quality colleagues at Eli Lilly and Company for their collaboration and dedication. In particular, I wish to acknowledge the contributions of Bill Chiasson, Rick Justice, Jole Rodriguez, and Irv Taylor.

Martin D. Hynes III

Contents

Contributors

Anthony C. Celeste   President, AAC Consulting Group, Inc., Bethesda, Maryland

Martin D. Hynes III   Director, Pharmaceutical Projects Management, Lilly Research Laboratories, Eli Lilly and Company, Indianapolis, Indiana

Richard M. Justice, Jr.   Group Leader, Quality Assurance—Clinical Trial Materials, Eli Lilly and Company, Indianapolis, Indiana

Arthur N. Levine   Partner, Arnold & Porter, Washington, D.C.

Robert A. Nash   Associate Professor of Industrial Pharmacy and Cosmetic Science, St. John's University, Jamaica, New York

Christopher T. Rhodes   Department of Applied Pharmaceutical Sciences, University of Rhode Island, Kingston, Rhode Island

Tara V. Sams   Director, Quality Management, Applied Analytical Industries, Inc. (AAI), Wilmington, North Carolina

Peter D. Smith   Director, Compliance Services—International, KMI/Parexel, Inc., Altanta, Georgia and Rockville, Maryland

Ronald F. Tetzlaff   KMI/Parexel, Inc., Atlanta, Georgia and Rockville, Maryland

Elizabeth MacLennan Troll   Head of Clinical/Preclinical Compliance, Guilford Pharmaceuticals, Inc., Baltimore, Maryland

Paul E. Wray   President, International Pharmaceutical Services, Bridgewater, New Jersey

1

Introduction to Food and Drug Administration Pre-New Drug Applications Approval Inspections

Martin D. Hynes III
Eli Lilly and Company, Indianapolis, Indiana

I. DEFINITION OF A PRE-NEW DRUG APPLICATIONS APPROVAL INSPECTION

A. Inspection History

A pre-approval inspection is a visit by one or more food and drug investigators to review the adequacy and accuracy of the information provided in a regulatory submission (*Compliance Program Guidance Manual, Program 7346.832*). The program was first implemented in the Food and Drug Administration's (FDA's) mid-Atlantic region, which has the largest number of pharmaceutical manufacturing plants in the United States. Leadership for the program during its formative years was provided by Henry Avallone, Joe Phillips, and Richard Davis of the mid-Atlantic office. The first formal communication of the program was in a 1990 publication authorized by Henry Avallone entitled "Mid-Atlantic Region Pharmaceutical Inspection Program."

Shortly thereafter, a formal compliance manual was issued by the agency. This manual, entitled *The FDA Compliance Program Guidance Manual on Pre-Approval Inspections/Investigations* (*Program 7346.832*), was formally published in October 1990. The manual outlined a role for both the Center for Drug Evaluation and Research (CDER) and the Field or District Offices in the drug approval process, thus adding an additional review step to the new drug approval

1

process. The application for marketing approval was now to be reviewed for Good Manufacturing Practices (GMP) compliance as well as the adequacy and accuracy of the data provided in the submission. Before this time, data submitted in New Drug Applications (NDAs) and Approved New Drug Applications (ANDAs) were rarely, if ever, audited for authenticity and accuracy. Thus, for all intents and purposes, companies were on the honor system. With the advent of the generic drug scandal in the late 1980s, this all changed radically. The honor system was effectively terminated with the generic drug scandal. This was confirmed by Dr. David Kessler (then the commissioner of the FDA) in 1990, when he said "What I learned most from the generic drug scandal is that in the end, the data this agency acts on has to be audited. The honor system is out the window" [1].

It is doubtful that the FDA will ever reinstate the honor system that existed before the generic drug scandal of 1989, despite the fact that the results from pre-approval inspections have gotten significantly better over the past several years. This level of improved performance is evidenced by the fact that the FDA recommendations to withhold approval have declined significantly over the past 7 years from a 1990 high of 60% to less than 30% in 1996, even though the number of inspections has increased.

The pre-approval inspection program has evolved over the past several years (Figure 1). Understanding the evolution of this program over time is essential to designing and implementing a program within your company to successfully prepare for an FDA pre-approval inspection. Despite the fact that the history of the pre-approval inspection started with the generic drug scandal and the appointment of Dr. David Kessler as commissioner of the FDA, one needs to go back to the late 1970s to fully understand the program and its implications.

In September of 1978, the preamble to the current GMP (cGMP) was published in the *Federal Register*. The part of the preamble that is relevant to the pre-NDA approval inspection program reads as follows:

> The commissioner finds that as stated in 211.1 these cGMP regulations apply to the preparation of any drug product for administration to humans or animals, including those still in investigational stages. It is appropriate that the process by which a drug product is manufactured in the development phase be well documented and controlled in order to assure the reproducibility of the product for further testing and for ultimate commercial production. The Commissioner is considering proposing additional cGMP regulations specifically designed to cover drugs in research stages [2].

Embedded in this short statement from the preamble to the cGMP are two important concepts that provide the underpinning of the entire pre-NDA approval inspection program.

The first concept is that the FDA has jurisdiction over drug products that are in clinical trials before approval. Thus, to the FDA, compliance to cGMP in the

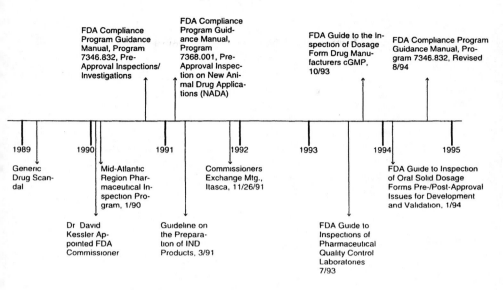

Figure 1 FDA Pre-NDA approval inspection: FDA time line.

manufacture of clinical trial materials was a well-established principle at the time the pre-approval inspections were enacted in the early 1990s.

The second concept that was established in the preamble to the cGMP was that the regulations for clinical trial materials were different for those that applied to the production of commercial products. This is evidenced by the fact that the FDA was considering proposing additional cGMP to cover drugs in the research stages.

To date, the FDA has elected not to issue cGMPs exclusively for investigational drugs. Rather, the agency has established its expectations through the issuance of various guidance documents, compliance programs, inspection guides, and podium policy presentations.

In addition, the preamble to the cGMP, the draft Guideline on the Preparation of Investigational New Drug (IND) Products, which was issued in February 1988, provided additional guidance in the application of cGMP to clinical trial materials. The guidelines, which were formally published in March 1991, clearly stated that at the stage at which the drug was to be produced for clinical trials in humans, compliance to cGMP was required.

These IND guidelines emphasized the need for proper documentation during the drug development process. Additionally, they specifically addressed control of components, production controls, process controls, equipment identification, packaging, and labeling. They also indicated that tighter controls should be implemented as additional experience was gained with the product as it progresses through the various stages of clinical development.

Thus, between the GMP preamble and the IND regulations, the FDA had firmly established its jurisdiction over materials produced for clinical trials before the generic drug scandal of 1989.

The Mid-Atlantic Region Pharmaceutical Inspection Program was the first of various documents issued by the FDA with the intention of educating the compliance branch of the FDA as well as the industry regarding the FDA's expectations. The two compliance documents that formalized the principles outlined in the Mid-Atlantic Region Pharmaceutical Inspection Program and issued by the FDA are as follows:

(1) *FDA Compliance Program Guidance Manual, on Pre-Approval Inspections/Investigations* (*Program 7346.832*), October 1990.
(2) *FDA Compliance Program Guidance Manual, on Pre-Approval Inspection of New Animal Drug Applications* (*NADA*) (*Program 7368.001*), February 1991.

B. Objectives of the Program

The objectives of this program can be summarized as follows:

(1) Ensure that facilities listed have the capabilities to fulfill the application commitments to manufacture, process, control, package, and label a drug product following GMP.
(2) Ensure adequacy and accuracy of analytical methods by proper testing.
(3) Ensure correlation between manufacturing process for clinical trial material, bioavailability study material, and stability studies and filed process.
(4) Ensure that scientific evidence supports full-scale production procedures and controls.
(5) Have submitted factual data.
(6) Ensure protocols are in place to validate the manufacturing process.

C. Role of CDER Versus the District Office

The FDA Compliance Program Guidance Manual (*Program 7346.832*) was revised in August 1994. That revision provides improved guidance for all phases of the inspection, sample collection, laboratory evolution, and assessment of findings. Additionally, the revisions to Program 7346.832 outline the roles for the CDER and the District Offices in the inspection process. The CDER's role was defined as reviewing the data submitted as a part of the NDA and generic applications and establishing the specifications for the product, whereas the role for the District Office was to audit the data for both authenticity and accuracy; determine the adequacy of the facilities, personnel, and equipment; and ensure cGMP compliance. A more detailed list of items to be reviewed and the role of the CDER and the District Office is provided in Table 1.

The CDER also has the role of assigning pre-approval inspections in the following cases: (1) narrow therapeutic range; (2) new chemical entities; (3) generic versions of the 200 most prescribed drugs; (4) drugs that are difficult to manufacture; (5) drugs that represent a new dosage form for the application; (6) first approval for the company; and (7) a poor GMP track record.

Once the agency has elected to conduct an inspection, they will place emphasis on the following areas during the conduct of that inspection: (1) compliance with cGMP; (2) documentation of bioequivalence; (3) bioavailability and stability studies; (4) the scientific evidence that supports the scale-up to production; and (5) the accuracy of information that is filed versus found. A detailed review of cGMP compliance and its relationship to pre-approval inspections is covered in Chapter 11.

Table 1 The Compliance Program on Pre-Approval Inspections/Investigations (7346.832)

Items to be reviewed	CDER	District
Biobatch manufacture	X	X
Manufacture of drug substance	X	X
Manufacture of excipients	X	X
Raw materials—cGMP		X
Raw materials (tests, methods, specifications)	X	X
Finished dosage form	X	X
Container/closure systems	X	X
Labeling and packaging controls		X
Labeling and packaging materials	X	
Laboratory support of methods validation	X	X
Product controls	X	X
Product test methods and specifications	X	X
Product stability	X	X
Comparison of pre-approval batches to commercial	X	X
Facilities, personnel, and equipment qualification		X
Process validation	X	X
Reprocessing	X	X
Ancillary facilities	X	X

II. AREAS OF FOCUS DURING THE CONDUCT OF THE INSPECTION

To assess the areas previously mentioned, the FDA inspectors focus on the following areas during the course of the inspection: (1) the manufacturing process; (2) validation; (3) reprocessing; (4) laboratory units; (5) components; (6) buildings and facilities; (7) equipment; (8) packaging and labeling controls; (9) sample collection; and (10) history of the development report.

A. The Manufacturing Process

The FDA inspectors assess the filed manufacturing process by auditing all facilities, equipment, procedures, and controls to ensure that they are ready to perform as specified in the application. The documentation from the facilities and controls used to make the biobatch/clinical batches are also the subject of FDA scrutiny. A detailed list of documents that may be reviewed by the FDA is discussed in Chapter 8. The process used to make these clinical trial lots is compared with the process filed in the NDA to assess the level of similarity. The role of technology transfer is described in Chapter 9. Any batch record may be reviewed during the inspection. However, the most probable lot documentation to be reviewed is stability, biobatch validation, scale-up, and launch.

B. Validation

1. Bulk Drug Substance

Domestic Sites. The FDA expects the validation of bulk drug substance to be complete at the time of the pre-approval inspection, which would imply the completion of three lots at product scale to be manufactured and assayed by the time of the inspection. Emphasis is placed on the final step of the production process and other critical steps. Additionally, the FDA requires the validation of cleaning and analytical methods. The role that validation plays in pre-approval inspections is discussed in Chapter 7.

International Sites. The FDA also expects that the bulk drug substance be validated at the time of the inspection. Further details of the FDA expectations for international sites can be found in Chapter 3.

2. Drug Product

Domestic Sites. The validation of sterile or nonsterile drug products is not required at the time of the pre-approval inspection. However, the protocol for validation of the drug product should be available at the time of the inspection.

Experience with one full-scale lot at the site of manufacture is most beneficial at the time of inspection. In fact, many firms elect to run three lots, with the expectation that it will facilitate the approval process, and take the business risk that the materials will have expired by the time of approval. The role of validation in pre-approval inspection is addressed in Chapter 7.

International Sites. The validation of drug products, both sterile and non-sterile, should be completed before the FDA inspection. Further details on the FDA's expectations for foreign sites can be found in Chapter 3.

C. Reprocessing

All processes for reprocessing drug products must be included in the regulatory submission. The FDA inspects processes that have been included in the submission to ensure that the process has been validated and that the material derived from the reprocessing procedure is bioequivalent.

D. Laboratory Units

The inspectors from the FDA can be expected to evaluate laboratory facilities, training procedures, personnel, and equipment maintenance records. The accuracy and authenticity of the data generated in the laboratories that support both product development and manufacturing of commercial product may be checked by the FDA. The FDA expects to see laboratory equipment qualified and laboratory methods validated.

E. Components

The suppliers of active drug substances must be identified in the regulatory submission. These suppliers may also be inspected by the FDA as a part of the pre-approval inspection process. In the event that multiple suppliers are included, the firm needs to be able to prove bioequivalence of the materials produced by these different suppliers. If an excess of active ingredient is used in the commercial formulation, then data are required to support the use of the excess.

F. Buildings and Facilities

The FDA has the authority to inspect a wide range of facilities during the conduct of the pre-approval inspection. The facilities that may be inspected include any listed in the regulatory application or used during the development of the drug, and may include product development laboratories, analytical laboratories, bioequivalence testing laboratories, quality control laboratories, and facilities that manufacture clinical trial or commercial lots.

If the FDA elects to inspect these facilities, it assesses general cGMP compliance. The FDA also looks for the potential for cross-contamination with other drug products or clinical trial materials manufactured in the facility. The air handling and water systems may be inspected by the FDA during the course of the visit. The flow of people, equipment, and products through the facility may also be examined.

G. Equipment

The FDA inspectors expect to find the cleaning methods for the new drug substances and dosage forms at the time of the inspection. In all probability, these methods will not be validated until a later date. The firm needs to provide both installation qualification and operational qualification data for all of the equipment listed in the submission.

H. Packaging and Labeling Controls

During the course of the pre-NDA approval inspection, the FDA may very possibly review labeling and packaging controls. This review could encompass those in place for the labeling of clinical trial material as well as commercial product. Contract facilities involved in product labeling could also be the subject of an inspection. Copies of the draft product label should be available for the FDA inspectors.

I. Sample Collection

The FDA investigators conducting the pre-approval inspection have the authority to collect samples of the biobatch during the course of the pre-approval inspection. In the case of an ANDA, the FDA may collect samples of the companies' biobatch as well as samples of the innovator drug used as a comparator. These samples may be collected from the firm or the contract testing laboratory engaged in the conduct of these bioequivalent studies.

J. History of the Development Report

It is helpful to have copies of the history of the development report on hand for the FDA investigators during the course of the inspection. The purpose of this report is to summarize: (1) the experiments that were conducted to develop and select the manufacturing process used for the production of commercial product; and (2) the experimental evidence that ensures bioequivalence of production size lots to the lots used in clinical trials. The following types of information are generally contained in this report: (1) formulation; (2) types of equipment used; (3) manufacturing process; (4) in-process results; (5) final dosage form test results; (6) critical parameters of bulk drug substance; (7) conclusions with key variables identified; and (8) stability.

The history of the development report should be written on an ongoing basis during the development process. In this way, the report can be written in a chronological manner while the changes and accompanying rationale are still fresh in the scientist's mind. One such strategy is to update the history of the development report as each major milestone in the drug development process is achieved, such as the start of phase I, II, or III trials. In this way, the report does not have to be written at the end of the drug development cycle just before the FDA pre-approval inspection, when the memories of the changes that have occurred over a number of years have dimmed, the scientific talent may have changed, and there is intense time pressure to complete the report. Once the report is completed, it is best to have the document reviewed and approved by the management of the product development area, quality management, and the appropriate manufacturing site personnel (e.g., quality control, tech service).

III. CONCLUSIONS

This chapter provides a brief overview of FDA pre-approval inspections, covering both the definition of an inspection and the roles of the CDER and District Office, as well as outlining what the FDA inspectors will expect during the conduct of their inspection. The vast majority of the topics outlined here are covered in greater detail in the other chapters in this volume. This chapter provides an overview that will help in seeing the pre-approval inspection in a broad context and that will enhance the value of the subsequent chapters in this volume.

It is hoped that this chapter communicates at a high level the vast amount of information that is now known about FDA pre-approval inspections that has evolved over the first several years of the inspection program. Given the large number of areas that the FDA may inspect, it should be apparent that advanced preparation for the inspection is critical. Preparations of this magnitude cannot be successfully undertaken in the weeks and months before the inspection. Rather, the work of preparing for the inspection must be undertaken concurrently with the development of the drug. Chapter 2 outlines many of the preparation efforts that were used at Eli Lilly and Company to prepare for these inspections. Preparation of pre-approval inspections should be viewed as an ongoing drug development activity. The role of the quality assurance group in these preparation efforts is described in Chapter 11. Such a long-term view will greatly enhance the chances of passing the inspection and rapidly launching the product to patients in need. The consequences of failing a pre-approval inspection are outlined in Chapter 6. In addition to advanced preparation, it is imperative that the actual conduct of the inspection be well managed. Helpful hints on how to do this well are provided in Chapter 5.

REFERENCES

1. D. Kessler, *Medical Advertising News*, April 1991, pp. 23–25.
2. Human and Veterinary Drugs, Current Good Manufacturing Practices in Manufacture Processing, Planning and Holding, preamble to the current Good Manufacturing Practices (cGMP), Volume 43, No. 190, 1978, pp. 45014–45089.
3. Mid-Atlantic Region Pharmaceutical Inspection Program, *Inspection Guidance for Prescription Drug Plants*, 1990.
4. New Drug Evaluation Pre-Approval Audit Inspections, *The FDA Compliance Program Guidance Manual on Pre-Approval Inspections/Investigations (7346.832)*, 1994, previous edition 1990 (ID FDA 06698 and 06750).
5. *Guidelines on the Preparation of Investigational New Drug (IND) Products (Human and Animal)*, 1991.
6. Pre-Approval Inspection of New Animal Drug Applications (NADA), *FDA Compliance Program Guideline Manual, Program 7368.001*.

2

Developing a Strategic Approach to Preparing for a Successful Pre-NDA Approval Inspection

Martin D. Hynes III
Eli Lilly and Company, Indianapolis, Indiana

I. INTRODUCTION

The Food and Drug Administration (FDA) introduced pre–New Drug Applications (NDA) approval inspections in the early 1990s as a result of the generic drug scandal of the late 1980s. During the implementation of this program, a significant number of applications were turned down as a result of Good Manufacturing Practices (GMP) problems. In fact, in the first year, the turn-down rate was 60%. This high turn-down percentage had a significant impact on the pharmaceutical industry, prompting many companies to begin internal preparation efforts in anticipation of these GMP inspections. Initially these efforts had a short-term focus in that they were designed to prepare for FDA inspections that were likely to occur within the near term. At the same time, many companies also began to think about preparation on an ongoing basis over the course of the entire drug development cycle. Given the comprehensive nature of an FDA pre-NDA approval inspection and the magnitude of the preparation effort required to ensure a successful outcome, preparation cannot be effectively completed in a short period of time. This substantiates the need to incorporate pre-approval inspection preparation efforts into the ongoing drug development process. Such an ongoing investment is warranted if one considers the potential negative ramifications of not passing an FDA pre-approval inspection. The negative ramifications include, most importantly, the delayed introduction of new pharmaceuticals that offer significant therapeutic benefit to patients who are not well served by existing therapies as well as a significant loss of revenue for the pharmaceutical company submitting the application. Therefore, a significant degree of effort is warranted on the part of those participating in development of the drug to establish the internal drug development and business practices that will ensure a successful pre-approval inspection outcome.

This chapter describes a strategic approach to establishing internal drug development and business practices that will ensure preparedness for FDA pre-approval inspections.

II. STRATEGY DEVELOPMENT

Effective leadership and management are important dimensions in the running of any business. Leadership is of particular importance in a business where there is a high degree of change and complexity [1]. Additionally, leadership, employee involvement, customer focus, measurement, and improvement are key elements of a quality program. An excellent example of the role of leadership in a quality program within the context of a complex business undergoing significant change is illustrated in developing a strategy for pre-approval inspections. Leadership is of particular importance in the preparation for an FDA pre-approval inspection because it is required for the establishment of strategic direction and management of a complex business undergoing significant change. Once that direction is established, the goal is to align people behind that direction while motivating and inspiring them to work toward achieving the stated strategy. In the establishment of strategic direction, it is imperative that those in a leadership position listen to the voice of the customer, the business, and the best. The information obtained from listening to these three voices should be integrated by the leadership team for product development into a pre-approval inspection strategy that is unique for the product development organization. These three voices are first discussed separately so that their requirements can be fully understood. However, they ultimately must be integrated into one single unified unique strategy for the product development organization.

A. Voice of the Customer

The development of innovative new pharmaceuticals requires the approval of the FDA before they can be delivered to the ultimate customers (medical professionals and patients). Therefore, the FDA should be considered a customer of the product development organization. Thus, in the formulation of a pre-approval strategy, the valid requirements of the FDA need to be understood and incorporated. These requirements include those that apply during the development period as well as those at the time of marketing approval. As we consider the requirements of the FDA, there are general customer criteria that are important to keep in mind. These general criteria suggest that customer requirements should be reasonable, understandable, measurable, believable, and achievable. Within the context of these criteria, the FDA's requirements for the manufacture of clinical trial materials indicate "when drug development reaches the stage where the drug products are produced for clinical trials in humans and animals, then compliance with the cGMP is required" [2]. The FDA's requirements have evolved and become much more explicit since the IND guidelines were issued in draft form in 1988. The evolution of these requirements over time is shown in Figure 1. The origin of the pre-approval inspection program can be traced back to the Mid-Atlantic Region Drug Inspection Program, which was issued in January 1990 [3]. The pre-approval inspection program was formally implemented in March 1990. *The FDA Compliance Program Guidance Manual on Pre-Approval Inspections/Investigations (Program 7346.832)* was officially issued in October 1990 [4]. A revised version of this compliance manual was then issued in August 1994.

The pre-approval inspection *Compliance Program Guidance Manual* delineates how and when the FDA will inspect to ensure that its valid customer requirements are met. The FDA's Center for Drug Evaluation and Research (CDER) has required FDA field investigators to conduct pre-approval inspections for the

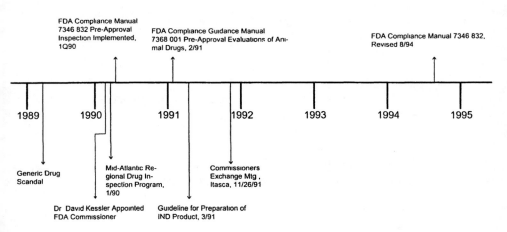

Figure 1   FDA Pre-NDA approval inspection guidelines over time.

following types of drugs: new chemical entities, those with a narrow therapeutic range, and the generic versions of the 200 most prescribed drug or drugs that are difficult to manufacture. They have also required inspections for firms that have a poor GMP track record, firms that are requesting their first ever approval, or those that are requesting approval for a drug formulation that they had not previously manufactured.

The object of these inspections is to ensure that the development/manufacturing facilities listed in the new drug application have the capabilities to manufacture, process, control, package, and label a drug product in compliance with the current GMP (cGMP). The inspection program also seeks to ensure the adequacy of analytical methods by proper testing and the validation of the manufacturing process. An additional objective is to investigate the correlation between the process used for the production of clinical trial materials, bioavailability study materials, and stability studies with the process filed in the NDA. This provides a degree of assurance to the FDA that sound scientific evidence supports the full-scale production procedures and controls proposed by the firm filing the NDA.

B. Voice of the Business

The requirements of the FDA should appropriately have a significant impact on the development of a strategic direction for the product development organization. However, other sources of input have to be taken into consideration; one of these is the voice of the business. The business of developing new products is perhaps the most complex process that any corporation undertakes [5]. This is particularly true when one considers the complexity of development of new chemical entities for the treatment of unmet medical needs. This task is not only complex but also exceedingly expensive and risky. Drug development costs have risen over the past several decades [6], while the overall success rate has decreased [7]. During the time that the FDA has been implementing the pre-approval inspection program, the pharmaceutical industry has seen profound changes. These changes have been seen in both the regulatory and business environment. In addition to the advent of pre-approval inspection programs, other regulatory changes have included the introduction of GCP (Good Clinical Practices) in Japan and the omnibus adverse event reporting requirements here in the United States. The advent of the FDA's new fraud policy and Disbarment Act indicates that the FDA is applying more scrutiny than ever to the data that go into new drug applications. While the compliance regulatory expectations have increased over the past 5 years, economic conditions impacting the pharmaceutical industry have also undergone profound change. This is evidenced by an increase in therapeutic and generic substitution in an environment that is moving toward managed health care. The most important of all these business drivers is the patient. Despite significant advances in the last 50 years, many diseases are still not well treated by modern pharmaceuticals. Thus, many patients are still waiting for new drug therapies to treat/cure their medical conditions, and patients are becoming strong advocates for the development of effective drug therapies. This is evidenced by the impact of the acquired immunodeficiency syndrome (AIDS) activists on the development of new drugs for the treatment of AIDS. These business drivers, when taken together, suggest that there has been significant change within the pharmaceutical industry. Given the complexity of the business, this suggests that considerable leadership and management skills are called for in the formulation and implementation of a strategy to ensure successful FDA pre-approval inspections.

C. Voice of the Best

In the development of strategic direction for pre-approval inspections, it is important to learn from the voice of the best. Many firms have had significant experience with pre-approval inspections. It is important to learn from their experiences, both good and bad. Many important lessons can be garnered by reading the other chapters in this volume. Additionally, it is possible through freedom of information to gain insight into the results of the most recent FDA pre-approval inspections. Use of freedom of information on an ongoing basis will allow your firm to keep abreast of the most up-to-date trends and FDA expectations. Benchmarking with other firms is yet another way to see how other pharmaceutical companies are preparing for pre-approval inspections.

D. Integration

Gathering information from these three voices provides the data needed to develop a rational strategy. Integrating these various inputs into a unique strategy for your drug development unit is the next step in the process of strategy development. It is important to note that it is not possible or prudent to take the strategy of another firm and try to directly implement it in your firm. This is particularly true as the data from these three voices may be different for each firm. Additionally, the business process and internal functional area responsibilities differ from firm to firm, thereby making it imperative that each organization develops its own unique strategy that is tailor-made for their organization. This unique strategy must fit within the overall drug development and corporate strategies that exist to guide the organization. Thus, pre-approval strategy must also be strongly linked to the organization's overall business strategy and drug development strategy. Once this strategy has been developed, it must be widely communicated throughout the research and development organization. The communication strategy must stress the fit of the pre-approval strategy within the context of the firm's overall strategy and its drug development strategy. Once the strategy has been developed and communicated, progress in its implementation must be measured on an ongoing basis.

III. SHORT- AND LONG-TERM STRATEGIC APPROACHES TO PREPARATION EFFORTS

The strategy that emerged from our internal efforts at Eli Lilly and Company contained two key elements. These elements were of a temporal nature in that both short- and long-term strategies were developed in response to the FDA implementation of the pre-NDA approval inspection program. These short- and long-term efforts are depicted in Figure 2. The short-term strategy was designed to guide our preparation efforts for a pre-approval inspection in the months and weeks before its scheduled occurrence.

A. Short-Term Strategic Approaches

This strategy contained 10 preparation steps that are believed to lead to a successful inspection outcome. These 10 steps are listed in Table 1 and have been described in detail by Justice et al. [8] of Lilly Research Laboratories. The first step of this preparation program is to determine the state of cGMP compliance of all of the manufacturing and development facilities listed in the NDA for the

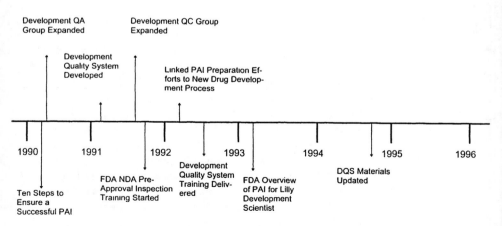

Figure 2   FDA Pre-NDA approval inspections time line: the Lilly response.

Table 1 Ten Steps to a Successful Pre-NDA Approval Inspection

1. Determine state of cGMP compliance
2. Compile regulatory documents
3. Prepare Regulatory Commitment Document (RCD)
4. Identify key batch records
5. Compare key batch records to regulatory documents
6. Write analytical methods history review
7. Transfer analytical methods (i.e., site certification)
8. Review analytical raw data
9. Scale-up in preparation for launch materials
10. Write development report (new drug dosage form/bulk drug substance)

product under review. The quality assurance organization for development has the responsibility of conducting these assessments. Secondly, all of the appropriate regulatory documents are compiled for use by the FDA inspectors at the potential inspection sites. Additionally, the regulatory commitments made by the firm to the FDA in these documents are summarized by the regulatory affairs group into one user-friendly summary document. The fourth step in preparing for a successful pre-NDA approval inspection is the identification of key batch records. These documents are then compared (step five of the process) with the commitments that are contained in the Regulatory Commitment Document. Any discrepancies identified are resolved, and explanations are documented when appropriate. Steps four and five are undertaken by the product development scientists in collaboration with the quality control and regulatory affairs departments. The history of analytical methods used to control the product is prepared as part of step six of the process. The analytical development department prepares a chronological history of the analytical methods used throughout the development time line. Included in this document are the justifications for any and all changes made in the methods during the development process. As a part of this step, the analytical development scientist compares the methods used to release each batch of clinical trial material against the analytical methods in the regulatory documents applicable at the time of release. The seventh step in this preparation process is the transfer of analytical methods (i.e., site certification). At this time, the analytical development division transfers each one of the methods from the development site where the assay was developed to sites that will use them for release of commercial products. The review of the analytical raw data is the eighth step in the preparation effort. The goal of this step is to ensure that the data are readily accessible to the FDA inspectors. Once the data have been compiled, the development scientist reviews the raw data of the "key" batches to ensure their completeness.

Step nine of this 10-step inspection preparation process is the scale-up in preparation for launch. At this point in time, installation qualification/operational qualification/performance qualification (IQ/OQ/PQ) activities are conducted. These include cleaning validation, process validation, sterilization validation, etc., according to established corporate procedures. The tenth and final step is the writing of the history of the development report. This report has two main sections: one that addresses the new drug dosage form and one that deals with the bulk drug substance. The product development scientist compiles the scientific evidence in this report that demonstrates bioequivalency for the first clinical trial lot through those lots that will be used for launch. The process development scientist compiles the scientific evidence in a report that describes the evolution of the process over time in a reader-friendly document. A description of the current process is included along with a description of the chemical/physical characteristics, purity, related substances, specifications, and stability of the drug substance.

To ensure that these steps are performed, an accountability matrix was developed. This matrix was designed to show each of the 10 steps along with the people who had primary responsibility for their initiation and timely completion. Additionally, the groups or departments involved as participants in the steps are also included. Table 2 shows the matrix for each of the 10 steps that was developed for Eli Lilly and Company.

B. Long-Term Strategic Approaches

The long-term strategy of preparing for a pre-NDA approval inspection is comprised of two important elements. The first is the integration of the pre-approval inspection into the process of drug development, and the second is the construction of a development quality system to provide cGMP guidance in the manufacture and distribution of clinical trial material.

1. Incorporation of Pre-Approval Inspections into the Overall Development Process

The preparation for pre-approval inspections must be incorporated into the overall process of drug development. In this way, a proactive preparation effort can be coupled with a short-term reactive approach in preparing for an FDA inspection. For us, this meant incorporation of the FDA pre-approval inspection into our drug development process map. Mapping of our development process is a key part of our efforts to reduce our drug development cycle time to an average of 2500 days. The development clock starts with the formation of a cross-functional project team and ends with the successful launch in two thirds of the intended world markets. This map of our development process contains milestones and well-defined deliverables (Figure 3). The first process milestone in our drug development process is the construction of a global development plan for the new chemical entity (NCE). The global development plan is an integration of the plans provided by the different functions, such as medical, toxicology, metabolism, and product and process development. The product and process development plan must encompass good development practices that will ensure a successful pre-approval inspection. Thus, the plan for a successful pre-approval inspection is incorporated into the NCE-specific development plan from the earliest days of product development work (Figure 4).

Additionally, our process maps include such important milestones as the validation activities, methods transfer, and the inspection itself (Figure 5). Thus, pre-approval inspections are viewed as a normal part of the drug development process that are planned for and managed in the same way as other important development activities such as the start of phase I studies.

2. Development Quality System

The other key component of our long-term strategy is a GMP quality system that was specifically designed for the production and distribution of clinical trial material. Therefore, it is different from the product quality system (PQS) in place for the manufacturing areas (Figure 6). This system was developed through a collaboration among product development scientists, quality assurance, and quality control professionals. At a minimum, such a system needs to include the following topics: batch disposition, stability, process validation, training, deviations, notification to management, documentation, change documentation, and history of development (Table 3). These topics are covered in high-level policy documents within Eli Lilly and Company.

The following examples provide a high-level overview of some of the key elements of several of our cGMP policy documents for product development.

Stability. The stability guideline calls for the generation of stability data to support development activities, clinical trial material in use, expiry dating, and regulatory submissions. The analytical development laboratories have the responsibility of conducting the assays to provide the needed data. Product development, technical services, and quality control can submit samples to analytical development for evaluation. Regulatory affairs needs to ensure that the studies meet the requirements of the appropriate regulatory agencies. Quality control plays a critical role in the review of nonconforming data.

Deviations. The development quality system contains a policy on the management of deviations. This policy requires that all deviations that impact clinical trial material be evaluated, justified, documented, and disposed of. These

Table 2 Pre-Approval Inspection Activity Matrix

No.	Activity	QA	CMC teams	Site cont.	Pharm. regulatory affairs	Tech. serv.
1	State of cGMP compliance	X	X	X		
2	Compile regulatory documents				I	
3	Prepare the RCD				I	
4	Identify the "key" batch records	X				X
5	Review conformance of key batch records to the RCD				X	X
6	Write analytical methods history review	X				
7	Transfer analytical methods					
8	Review analytical raw data					
9	Scale-up for preparation of launch materials					I
10	Write the development report					

I, initiator; X, participant; RCD, regulatory commitment document; QA, quality assurance; CT, clinical trial

deviations may be from standard operating procedures, development tickets, packaging orders, material specifications, analytical control procedures, and/or equipment maintenance schedules. Under this system, deviations can and should be reported by any employee involved in the manufacture of clinical trial material. However, the role of ensuring that appropriate action is taken after the deviation is reported rests with the quality control department that supports the product development organization.

Batch Disposition of Clinical Trial Lots. A quality system for product development should include a standard for disposition of clinical trial batches. Within our organization, the primary responsibility for clinical trial batch disposition rests with the quality control organization for product development, which is separate from the quality control organization that supports the manufacture of commercial drug products. The development quality control organization has the explicit responsibility of ensuring that the clinical trial material meets all applicable requirements. Additionally, they evaluate any deviations from these standards and ensure their proper documentation. After quality control approval the regulatory affairs group reviews the batch records against the Investigational New Drug (IND) and its amendments to ensure that all regulatory requirements

Analytical development	Analytical support for CT	Development scientist	Quality control	Site quality control laboratories	Stability quality control laboratories	Stability requirements	Validation
		X	I				
	X	X	I				
I			X	I			
I				X	X	X	
I		X		X	X	X	
			I	X			X
		I					

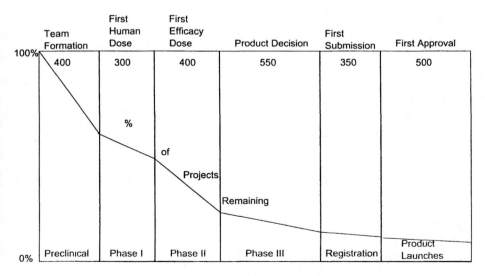

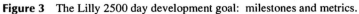

Figure 3 The Lilly 2500 day development goal: milestones and metrics.

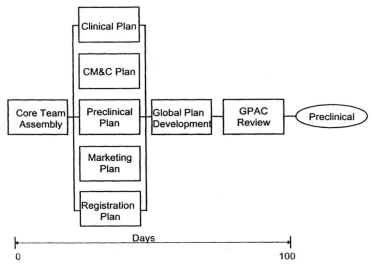

The CM&C plan contains the detailed plan for ensuring a successful pre-approval inspection.

Activity	Function	Deliverable
Core project team	Cross-functional	Integrated global development
Clinical plan	Medical	Plan for Phase I, II, and III clinical trials
CM&C plan	Product and process development	Functional plan for chemistry, manufacturing, control activities including pre-NDA approval inspection

Figure 4 Drug development process map: global plan development.

have been met before distribution to clinical trial investigators. The product development and analytical data needed to support these reviews are provided by product development and analytical groups.

Change Documentation. Another critical important part of a quality system for product development is the management change. The requirements for change documentation and management are articulated in a policy document. The focus is on changes that have the potential to impact safety, identity, strength, quality, or purity. This procedure is different from its counterpart in the manufacturing environment. This difference is driven by the fundamental difference in the nature of these two operations. The goal of the manufacturing area is to directly follow the manufacturing process that was developed by the product

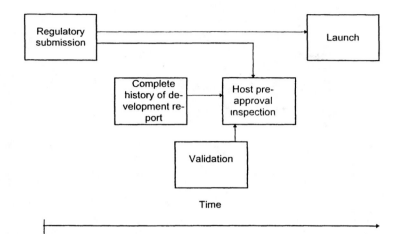

Figure 5 Drug development process map: pre-approval inspection.

Activity	Function	Deliverable
Regulatory submission	Regulatory	NDA submission
History of development report	Product and process development	A complete report with management approval
Validation	Development and manufacturing	A validated process/3 lots
Host pre-approval inspection	Quality assurance	Host FDA for duration of the inspection

development scientist and approved in the NDA, while the goal of the product development organization is to deliver a robust, efficient, and validated process to manufacturing. The development of this type of robust process requires extensive product development work throughout the development cycle. Change is an integral part of product development; therefore, it is important not to constrain or control change in the drug development process, but rather to document it and provide appropriate review and justification. This documentation provides the necessary input for regulatory changes, IND update, and amendments. Additionally, it provides background material for the history of the development document.

Process Validation. Given the importance of validation, from both the pre-approval inspection and business standpoints, it is an important part of any

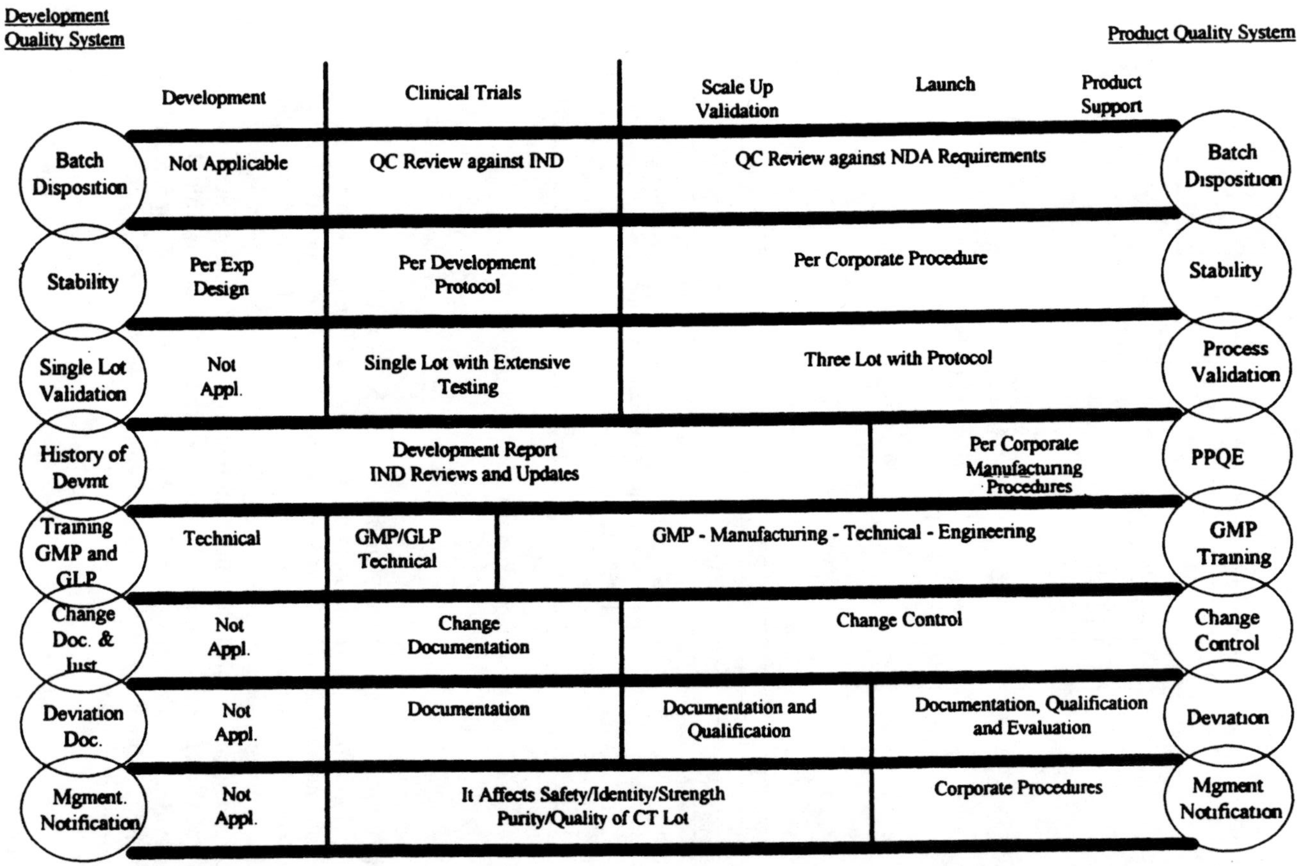

Figure 6 A comparison of the quality system for product development (DQS) to that for pharmaceutical products (PQS).

Table 3 Key Elements of a Development Quality System (DQS)

A quality system for product development should cover the following topics:

Batch disposition	Management notification
Stability	Documentation
Process validation	Change documentation
Training	History of development
Deviations	

development quality system. The operational definition of validation used in our quality system is the scientifically sound and documented evidence that each clinical trial lot will yield a product meeting all quality and design specifications. The development scientists in the product development area have the primary responsibility for developing the manufacturing process. This includes improving the process over time and documenting the changes made, including the necessary rationale and justification to support these changes. "Manufacturing" tickets used in the development area for the production of clinical trial lots are prepared by the scientist in concert with the clinical trial operations group. The goal is to provide clear process instructions and sampling rationale. This quality system procedure outlines a role for quality control and regulatory affairs in the review and approval of all process validation lots.

Training. Training is an integral part of any quality program. It is imperative that employees have adequate education and instruction so that they can perform their jobs according to established procedures and in accordance with the cGMP. A training procedure therefore represents an integral part of the development quality system. Its goal is to capture and institutionalize the corporate standard for training within the product development organization. The procedure calls for each employee to have a training plan that includes not only cGMP training, but also training on all applicable procedures, job skills, and transferable skills. The quality assurance group has the responsibility for the design, development, and delivery of cGMP and pre-approval training.

Management Notification. The procedure for management notification is an important element in the quality system for product development activities. This procedure sets the standard for notification of corporate research management in the event that a quality issue occurs with clinical trial materials within our organization. A person who becomes aware of a clinical trial material quality issue has the responsibility of notifying their management or the quality control group for clinical trial material. The quality control group has the explicit responsibility of assessing the potential risk associated with the identified issue by involving the appropriate experts from medical, development, toxicology, and quality assurance departments. The quality assurance group for product development has the explicit responsibility of determining if regulatory notification is required and the coordination of stock recovery actions when warranted.

History of Development Document. Given the importance of the history of development documents to the successful completion of a pre-approval inspection, a corporate standard has been incorporated into the development quality system. This procedure describes the content requirements for this document, which is designed to describe the history of product development from preliminary studies through regulatory submission. The product development scientist has the primary responsibility for authoring this document. The goal is to have this document updated on a regular basis so that it is always available for FDA inspection.

Topics other than those described here can and should be included in a development system for product development. The important thing is for each organization to have a quality system tailored to their organization that captures how they will comply with cGMP during drug development. Such a system will ensure that the organization is well prepared for a pre-approval inspection and minimizes the efforts needed just before the inspection itself.

IV. FOCUS ON IMPROVEMENT

Once a research organization has the fundamental building blocks needed to consistently pass pre-approval inspections, cGMP for drug development and development plans that incorporate pre-approval inspections, a formalized process is needed to continue to improve the system. Such a system will lead to a sustainable competitive advantage for the organization, which will be evidenced by a continual high degree of successes on pre-approval inspections. The establishment of such a system of continuous improvements will keep policies and procedures at a state of the art. Such a system should be built on the plan-do-check-act cycle (Figure 7). An improvement process of this nature was outlined in the 14 points of Dr. W. Edwards Deming in *A Theory for Management* [9]. Thus, the development of a systematic approach for the identification and resourcing of improvement projects can be translated into a competitive advantage: a consistently high rate of successful pre-approval inspections over time.

Over the past 6 years that the pre-approval inspection program has existed, it has gone through several changes and iterations. A systematic approach to improvement will help to ensure that the rate of internal change exceeds that in the external environment.

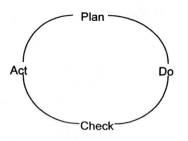

Figure 7 Quality improvement process: P-D-C-A cycle.

The identification of key issues in the product development process is essential to a focused and systematic improvement effort. These issues can be identified in a number of different ways. Several excellent sources came from the results of internal quality assurance audits, external audits conducted by the FDA, deviations, and periodic product quality evaluations (PPQE). The issues identified by these various techniques can be integrated into one overall list of areas for improvement. This singular list can then be prioritized using a variety of different criteria (Figure 8). Factors such as feasibility, potential return, impact across several development areas, degree of improvement possible, and amount of organizational pain associated with the issues can be used in the prioritization process. Projects that receive high priority can then be selected as improvement targets. Once an issue has been selected, a cross-functional/multidisciplinary team should be constituted to work on the issues. These improvement teams are resourced with expertise from organizational effectiveness, quality control, quality assurance, and the appropriate product development areas as appropriate to the problem or identified issues. The teams are given the responsibility to study the situation and make recommendations for improvement. These improvements are then institutionalized.

V. CONCLUSIONS

A successful pre-approval inspection program is key to bringing new drugs to the market in a timely manner for patients in need. A great deal of corporate leadership is needed to establish the strategic direction for an initial pre-approval inspection preparation effort, both in the short and long term. That effort must be based on an understanding of the voice of the business, the customer (FDA), and the experience of the best. The program must fit within an overall corporate

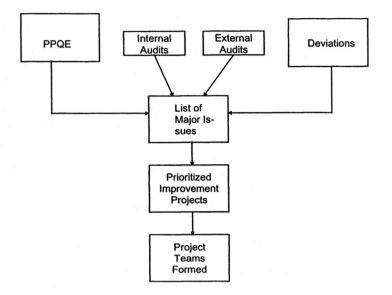

Figure 8 Improvement team formation: impact.

strategy as well as the drug development strategy. Planning for the inspection must start from the earliest stages of compound development. Internal policies and procedures must be in place to ensure compliance with cGMP throughout the product development life cycle. The preparation effort for a pre-approval inspection must be seen as an integral part of the development effort, not as a last-minute effort.

REFERENCES

1. J. P. Kotter, *A Force for Change: How Leadership Differs from Management*. The Free Press, New York, 1990.
2. *Guideline on the Preparation of Investigational New Drug Products (Human and Animal)*, March 1991.
3. *Mid-Atlantic Regional Drug Inspection Program*, January 1990.
4. *FDA Compliance Program Guidance Manual 7346.832 Pre-Approval Inspections/ Investigations*, October 1990, revised August 1994.
5. P. A. Roussel, K. N. Saad, and T. J. Erickson, *Third Generation R&D Managing. The Link to Corporate Strategy*. Harvard Business School Press, Arthur D. Little, Inc., Boston, 1991

6. J. A. DiMasi, R. W. Hansen, H. G. Grabowski, L. Lasagna, Research and Development Costs for New Drugs by Therapeutic Category. A Study of the US Pharmaceutical Industry, *PharmacoEconomics* 7:152–169 (1995).
7. J. A. DiMasi, Success Rates for New Drugs Entering Clinical Testing in the United States, *Clin. Pharmacol. Ther.* 58:1–14 (1995).
8. R. M. Justice, J. O. Rodriguez, W. J. Chiasson, Ten Steps to Ensure a Successful Pre-NDA Approval Inspection, *J. Parenteral Sci. Technol.* 47:89–92 (1993).
9. W. E. Deming, *Out of the Crisis*, Massachusetts Institute of Technology, Cambridge, Massachusetts, 1982.
10. *FDA Compliance Program Guidance Manual 7368.001 Pre-approval Evaluation of Animal Drugs*, February 1991.

3

Food and Drug Administration International Pre-Approval Inspections

Ronald F. Tetzlaff and Peter D. Smith
KMI/Parexel, Inc., Atlanta, Georgia and Rockville, Maryland

I. INTRODUCTION

A. Background

During the past few years, the Food and Drug Administration (FDA) has substantially increased the number of inspections under the international inspection program. For example, during fiscal year (FY) 1995, the FDA performed approximately 33% more drug inspections of offshore facilities than were accomplished in 1994 (380 versus 280, respectively). For FY 1996, the FDA performed a total of approximately 345 inspections at offshore pharmaceutical manufacturing and approximately 90 clinical study audits. A number of reasons account for this increase, including increased budget appropriations for the international program (e.g., Prescription Drug Use Free Act [PDUFA]), FDA concerns about the significant good manufacturing practices (GMP) violations that have been detected, and the FDA's reaction to the congressional oversight committee that has been investigating the international inspection program.

The FDA makes no distinction between international and domestic facilities when determining conformance with current GMPs (cGMPs). Another notable change during the past several years has been an increase in the degree of inspectional scrutiny at international sites under the FDA pre-approval inspection (PAI) program. In particular, more attention has been given to international manufacturers of finished pharmaceuticals and active pharmaceutical ingredients (APIs). Nearly 75% of the bulk active ingredients used in U.S. drug products are from international sources, and the majority of the international drug inspections (approximately 65%) cover APIs. The remaining 35% of the inspections cover dosage form manufacturers and audits of clinical studies or preclinical studies under good laboratory practices (GLPs). One consequence of the FDA's increased inspectional activity has been detection of conditions that do not conform to cGMPs. In fact, during FY 1995, 42% of the PAIs at international sites resulted in the FDA field office recommending withholding approval of applications. During FY 1996, the FDA field offices recommended withholding approvals at the rate of 24%.

The objective of this chapter is to describe some proactive steps that can be followed to make international inspections proceed as smoothly as possible. Specific objectives are as follows: (1) to present background and historical perspectives about the issues that have led up to the current program; (2) to describe the recent revisions to the organizational units that manage the FDA international inspection program; (3) to review effective techniques to prepare for international inspections; and (4) to present information about the FDA's international enforcement practices when it detects significant GMP deviations or application integrity issues are documented.

B. Historical Perspectives on International PAI

International PAIs are not new. In fact, for the past several decades, the FDA has had an active international inspection program where FDA investigators have inspected drug manufacturers in approximately 40 countries to determine conformance with cGMP regulations. The following is a brief summary of a few key events that led up to the current PAI program for international drug manufacturers.

The 1941 Insulin Amendment required the FDA to test the purity and potency of insulin, and in 1945, the Penicillin Amendment added the requirement for the FDA to test and certify the effectiveness of penicillin products. The FDA introduced a batch-by-batch certification program due to the highly variable potency of commercial batches. Subsequent amendments extended this requirement to all antibiotics. The FDA antibiotic certification program encompassed all antibiotics, including bulk pharmaceutical chemicals (BPCs) and finished pharmaceuticals. The intent of this program was not unlike the current PAI program in that it introduced provisions for the following:

(1) *Application review and approval*: Firms were required to submit original safety and efficacy data on FDA Form 5. The equivalent to current Abbreviated Antibiotic Drug Application (AADA) was a Form 6 that was used when safety and efficacy has already been established. The information filed in these applications was similar in content to the information

that is currently required to be filed in the chemistry, manufacturing, and control (CMC) section of a new drug application (NDA).

(2) *PAI*: The FDA initiated a program to conduct international inspections for the purpose of verifying commitments made in FDA Forms 5 and 6.

(3) *Certificates of analysis*: The FDA required firms to submit to the FDA certificates of analysis for each batch of antibiotic to be distributed in the United States (Form 7).

(4) *Sample analysis*: The FDA required firms to submit samples to the FDA laboratories for the agency to confirm conformance with regulatory specifications. A sample from each batch of antibiotic was sent to the FDA's National Center for Antibiotic Analysis testing in Washington, DC.

(5) *Fees for FDA services*: The FDA initiated a program to charge firms for the costs associated with FDA programming inspections and sample analysis under the antibiotic certification program.

(6) *FDA batch-by-batch release*: The FDA implemented a program to grant companies a formal release for each batch that was found by FDA analysis to meet specifications.

(7) *Annual re-inspection*: The FDA performed annual re-inspections of each antibiotic manufacturer, using certification fees to fund the expenses for domestic and international inspections.

The FDA antibiotic inspection program continued until 1983, when the program was abolished. In 1961, the FDA conducted its first international inspection of a nonantibiotic drug product after a U.S. manufacturer submitted a bid for a government contract where the source of bulk pharmaceutical was a European manufacturer. The inspection was conducted by Charles Wayne, an FDA inspector from the FDA's district office in New York City. Throughout the 1960s, the majority of international inspections were for antibiotics, funded by certification fees, and conducted jointly by headquarters and field personnel.

In the 1970s, the number of nonantibiotic drug inspections increased, with field personnel conducting most of the inspections. In fact, the early international inspections were managed by the FDA's New York district office before this function was transferred to FDA's headquarters in Rockville, MD. In 1971, the FDA formed a group in the Rockville, MD, office that was called the Foreign Inspection Staff. This early group coordinated with FDA reviewers and made assignments to FDA inspectors who resided in the FDA district offices and were members of the "foreign inspection cadre." During the early 1970s, the FDA established a cadre of national experts (NEs) who were assigned to the Foreign Inspection Staff and were stationed in FDA field offices. This was the FDA's earliest attempt to use senior investigators to perform foreign inspections. The original NEs were the first international and interdistrict inspectors and included the following FDA investigators: Charles Wayne (New York, NY), Richard E. Shepherd (Atlanta, GA), Philip Brodsky (Philadelphia, PA); James Buemiller (Chicago, IL); and Francis Barnes (Detroit, MI).

The first international medical device inspection was conducted in 1975. By the early 1980s, the FDA discontinued its antibiotic certification program (including terminating certification fees). At this point, the funding for the international inspection program was from the FDA's general budget. During the 1970s and early 1980s, the majority of inspections were for antibiotics, BPCs, and sterile injectable drugs. At that time, relatively few international inspections were performed at manufacturing sites of oral dosage forms or abbreviated NDA (ANDA) products.

In 1987, the FDA increased its budget for the international inspection program and began to conduct more international inspections. That year, the FDA's budget was approximately one quarter of a million dollars and approximately 180 inspections were conducted. In 1989 and 1990, the FDA began criminal investigations as a consequence of the generic drug scandal in the United States, when a number of individuals were found to have submitted false data in ANDA applications. The investigations found that a number of individuals had submitted fraudulent data and/or there were serious GMP deviations for a number of manufacturers of drugs covered by ANDA applications. These findings resulted in the FDA introducing an inspection program in 1990 (Compliance Program 7346.832) that provided for PAI inspections of each facility before the FDA would grant approval of NDA/ANDA applications. This program became to be known as the PAI program.

Since 1987, the numbers of international inspections has increased nearly every year (except during 1991, when international inspections were interrupted during the Gulf War). From the one quarter million dollar budget of 1987, the FDA has each year steadily increased its funding for international inspections to its current level (1997) of approximately 2 million dollars. In FY 1995, the FDA budget for international inspections peaked to its highest level at approximately $2.5 million, with approximately $750,000 to be used for PAIs from user fees being collected for the review of NDAs. The FY 1997 budget provides for approximately 2 million dollars for approximately 400 inspections of pharmaceutical manufactures, 500 inspections of medical device facilities, and 100 food manufacturers.

In addition to the international inspections of pharmaceuticals, the FDA also conducts international inspections of biologicals that are covered by Establishment License Application/Product License Application (ELA/PLA). The Center for Biologics Evaluation and Research (CBER) also conducts international PAIs. In 1993, the FDA began transferring the responsibility for inspections of international blood banks and some other biologics from CBER personnel to the field inspection cadre. Although CBER will retain inspectional responsibility for vaccines, most other biological products will be inspected either jointly with the CBER and field personnel or exclusively by investigators from FDA field offices. The funding for CBER inspections is covered by a separate FDA budget and CBER inspection programs.

II. FDA ORGANIZATIONAL RESPONSIBILITIES FOR INTERNATIONAL PAIs

To be effective in coordinating PAIs and to facilitate the NDA/ANDA review process, pharmaceutical company management needs to understand the roles and responsibilities of the various FDA units that are involved with managing the international inspection program.

The FDA currently has approximately 9000 employees located in various offices throughout the United States. The FDA has two major components: the headquarters and the field offices. Approximately one half of the employees are in FDA headquarter offices that are located in approximately 40 different office buildings in the Rockville, MD, area (near Washington, DC). The remainder of the employees are assigned to the district offices that are located in major U.S. cities. The FDA has no offices overseas.

A. FDA Headquarters Offices

The headquarters organization is divided into more components than can be described in this chapter. The following is a brief description of the key head-quarters and field units within the FDA that companies will most likely deal with during their preparations for a foreign PAI of drug products.

1. Office of Regulatory Affairs

The Office of Regulatory Affairs (ORA) is the headquarters unit that provides a management function for the various FDA field offices, including the district offices and specialized laboratories throughout the country. The ORA, headed by the Associate Commissioner for Regulatory Affairs, consists of a number of headquarters divisions and the entire field force, totaling approximately 3000 employees.

The ORA field investigators and analysts who perform foreign PAIs represent all districts (see Section II.A.2). At the completion of each foreign inspection where objectionable conditions or practices are detected, the investigators (and/or analyst) will issue to responsible management a written list of observations (FDA form FDA-483). Upon return to their local offices, the FDA team will prepare an Establishment Inspection Report (EIR), which is reviewed and endorsed by the investigator's field supervisor. The EIRs for international facilities are then forwarded to headquarters (CBER or Center for Drug Evaluation and Research [CDER]) for final review and disposition (see Section II.A.3).

2. Division of Emergency and Investigational Operations

The Division of Emergency and Investigational Operation (DEIO), originally formed in 1971 as the Foreign Inspection Staff, operated for the past decade as the International Technical Operations Branch (ITOB). In 1996, this unit was reorganized as part of a merger of two headquarters divisions (Division of Field Investigations [DFI] and the Division of Epidemiological and Emergency Operations [DEEO]). The newly created division is now called the DEIO. This unit has been the focal point for the foreign inspection program and is a source of technical assistance and guidance for the international and domestic companies. The DEIO provides investigative technical support functions and conducts reviews of facility design and construction for both domestic and international facilities. The FDA's NE cadre that was formerly assigned to the ITOB within the DFI has been reassigned to the DEIO. This new unit also provides specialized technical training for FDA personnel at district offices and for national training programs.

The DEIO is organized into six functional groups (Drugs, Devices, Foods, Biologicals, Emergency and Complaints, and Professional Support Services). Each group is responsible for both domestic and foreign activities within the respective commodity. There are three groups that have responsibilities for international PAIs, including drugs, biologics, and medical devices. The Drugs Group is responsible for managing and directing international inspections covering human drugs, veterinary drugs, and clinical/nonclinical study audits. The Devices Group is responsible for directing and managing medical device foreign inspections. The Biologicals Group coordinates with the CBER to accomplish inspections at foreign blood and blood products, and biological pharmaceutical manufacturers.

The DEIO includes a cadre of more than one dozen NEs who, as part of their normal activities, conduct international inspections. These individuals, who are expert investigators in at least one of FDA inspectional disciplines such as drugs, devices, sterile products, or computers, are located in FDA field offices and are attached to the various groups in the DEIO, receiving their work assignments from the DEIO group. The current cadre of NEs are listed in Table 1.

A primary role of the DEIO with regard to international inspections is to coordinate with the FDA district offices to obtain the cadre members to perform

Table 1   The Current Cadre of National Experts

Name	FDA district/specialty	Phone number
Thomas Arista	Dallas/Biotechnology	(214) 655-5308
David J. Bergeson	Kansas City/Computer	(316) 269-7165
Mary T. Carden	Buffalo/Biologics	(716) 846-4468
Karen A. Coleman	Atlanta/Devices	(404) 347-3218
Robert Coleman	Atlanta/Drugs, BIMO	(404) 347-3218
Debra Devlieger	Seattle/Food, LACF	(206) 553-7001
David L. Duncan	Detroit/Drugs, BIMO	(317) 226-6500
Mike Ellison	Baltimore/Food, LACF	(410) 749-0540
Charles M. Edwards	Philadelphia/Drugs, BIMO	(215) 597-0983
Joan A. Loreng	Philadelphia/Biologics	(215) 362-0740
David C. Pulham	Los Angeles/Drugs	(602) 379-4595
Joseph J. Stojak	Chicago/Devices	(708) 688-5462
Norman Wong	Seattle/Devices	(206) 483-4935

the international assignments that are issued from the respective centers. The DEIO is also responsible for notifying the companies of the planned inspection dates and for coordinating travel plans. The DEIO coordinates with international regulatory agencies and serves as a liaison between the various FDA offices and the international companies being inspected. The DEIO reviews responses received from companies after FDA international inspections, and makes recommendations for follow-up or proposes regulatory or administrative sanctions to the appropriate FDA office(s).

Companies that are uncertain about FDA procedures and policies for international inspections (or if they experience any difficulties) may contact the DEIO office for guidance. Table 2 lists the names, titles, and areas of responsibilities for key personnel that are currently in this office.

3. National Centers

The FDA, with the exception of the ORA, is organized into five centers that are based on product lines (Table 3). The centers promulgate regulations, develop inspection programs and guidance documents that are used by field offices, and review and approve enforcement actions that may be recommended by the field offices.

CDER.   Once an application (NDA/ANDA) has been accepted for filing by a CDER review division, a request for GMP status is sent to the Investigations and

Table 2 Key Personnel in the FDA DEIO Office

Food and Drug Administration
DEIO/Division of Emergency and Investigational Operations (HFC-130)
5600 Fishers Lane, Room 13-64
Rockville, MD 20857
Telephone: (301) 827-5653
Facsimile: (301) 443-6919

Drugs Group
  Manager: Mr. Jon Hunt
  Primary contact for foreign inspections: Ms. Deborah Browning; Ms. Rochelle Kimmel
  Telephone: (301) 827-5648; (301) 827-5663
  Facsimile: (301) 443-6919

Devices Group
  Manager: Irving Weitzman
  Primary contact for foreign inspections: Ms. Jaqueline Queen
  Telephone: (301) 827-5646
  Facsimile: (301) 443-6919

Biologicals Group
  Manager: Mr. John Hunt
  Primary contact for foreign inspections: Mr. Mark Hackman
  Telephone: (301) 827-5653
  Facsimile: (301) 443-6919

Table 3 The Five Centers of the FDA

Product type	Center
Drugs	Center for Drug Evaluation and Research (CDER)
Biologics	Center for Biologics Evaluation and Research (CBER)
Medical devices	Center for Devices and Radiological Health (CDRH)
Veterinary products	Center for Veterinary Medicine (CVM)
Foods and cosmetics	Center for Food Safety and Nutrition (CFSAN)

Pre-Approval Compliance Branch within the Division of Manufacturing and Product Quality at the CDER's Office of Compliance (Table 4). The Office of Compliance initiates an assignment for a PAI by sending a written assignment to the DEIO unit. The Office of Compliance is responsible for assuring that every manufacturing facility listed in each NDA/ANDA has been verified as being in compliance with cGMPs and has been determined to have the capability to perform the intended functions listed in the application. Such evaluations take place before the FDA grants approval to market the drug product.

The Investigations and Pre-Approval Compliance Branch is a national clearinghouse for PAI assignments. Review divisions extract manufacturing facility information from applications and request status reports from the Investigations and Pre-Approval Compliance Branch. The Investigations and Pre-Approval Compliance Branch then makes appropriate PAI assignments to domestic districts and the DEIO for foreign firms. Once a GMP status and clearance is received regarding each facility, the Investigations and Pre-Approval Compliance Branch makes a recommendation to the review division to either approve the application or withhold approval.

Several members of the Investigations and Pre-Approval Compliance Branch have been designated to form the Foreign Inspection Team. Since November 1994, this group has been charged with the responsibility to review the foreign EIRs, as well as EIRs for both foreign and domestic.

Table 4 Key Personnel in the CDER Office of Compliance

CDER Office of Compliance (HFD-300)
Metro Park North (MPN-1)
7520 Standish Place
Rockville, MD 20855
Director: Stephanie Grey

Division of Manufacturing and Product Quality (HFD-320)
   Director: Joseph Famulare
   Telephone: (301) 594-0093

Investigations and Pre-Approval Compliance Branch (HFD-324)
   Chief: Mark A. Lynch
   Telephone: (301) 827-0063
   Facsimile: (301) 594-2202

Foreign Inspection Team, Room 272 (HFD-322)
   Team Leader: John M. Dietrick
   Telephone: (301) 594-0095
   Facsimile: (301) 594-2202

Center for Veterinary Medicine. Pre-approval assignments to the field from the Center for Veterinary Medicine (CVM) are handled directly from the center to the domestic district offices or the DEIO. The pre-approval process and requirements for veterinary medical products are similar to those for human drug products. The contact personnel for the CVM is listed in Table 5.

CBER. For many years, domestic and foreign biologics inspections were conducted by staff from CBER's Rockville headquarters. Since the early 1990s, the ORA and CBER have engaged in a program to conduct joint ORA/CBER inspections at blood bank and biological pharmaceutical facilities, and in some cases the inspectional responsibilities have been completely absorbed by the ORA. Inspection of some CBER-regulated products, such as vaccines, will continue to be performed by CBER staff (Table 6).

B. FDA Field Offices and International Inspection Cadre

The FDA's international inspection cadre consists of approximately 500 employees from district offices that are located throughout the United States. Each district office has the responsibility for inspecting the regulated companies located within the geographical boundaries of the district. In each district office there are a number of resident post offices where one or more FDA investigator is stationed in various cities. Volunteers for the international inspection cadre are selected based on their experience. Cadre members have varied levels of experience, ranging from senior specialists with more than 20 years experience to individuals having as few as 4 or 5 years experience. Areas of specialization may include drugs, medical devices, and biologicals. Newly selected cadre members receive specialized training in international travel and FDA international operations either by attending a formal week-long FDA training course and/or by accompanying an experienced traveler on an initial trip.

The international inspections are performed by the NE cadre or by district investigators and analysts on temporary assignment. The duration of international trips are generally 3 or 4 weeks and included three to eight inspections depending

Table 5 CVM Contact Personnel

Contact:	Michael Smedley / HFV-102
	Center for Veterinary Medicine
	Metro Park North (MPN-2)
	7500 Standish Place
	Rockville, MD
	Telephone: (301) 594-1623
	Facsimile: (301) 594-2297

Table 6 CBER Office of Compliance

Director:
 Currently vacant (HFM-600)
 Telephone: (301) 594-2066

Foreign Inspections Contact:
 CBER Inspection Task Force (HFM-605)
 Telephone: (301) 594-0653
 Facsimile: (301) 594-1944

on the industry and the nature of the assignments. The *FDA/ORA Foreign Inspection and Travel Guide* contains instructions that are provided to the investigators and analysts who conduct foreign inspections (FDA, 1994). In 1996, the FDA published two Foreign Inspection Guides, one for drugs and one for medical devices (see Appendix 1).

III. PREPARING FOR INTERNATIONAL INSPECTIONS

A. Understanding International Inspection Procedures

In principle, FDA inspections are conducted in the same manner for either domestic or international firms, but in practice there are legal and logistical reasons for the FDA to follow different procedures when scheduling and conducting international inspections. The FDA has two main focuses when performing domestic and international inspections: (1) to verify integrity of information supporting applications made to the FDA; and (2) to determine conformance with GMPs. FDA inspections include a review and evaluation of the facilities, processes, and the product(s) to determine whether there are adequate assurances of identity, strength, quality, and purity.

Various publications describe the procedures and practices followed by the FDA during international inspections. Appendix 1, Selected FDA Guidelines, Guides, and Guidance Documents Related to PAIs, lists a number of key documents that describe issues that are likely to be addressed during PAIs.

1. Differences Between International and Domestic Inspections

There are four differences between domestic and international inspections that deserve mention: (1) international inspections are nearly always scheduled in advance; (2) language barriers pose unique challenges during international inspections; (3) international inspections are typically of shorter duration than domestic inspections that are conducted for the same purpose; and (4) typically, international firms are re-inspected less often than domestic facilities. The following describes some of the factors that account for the differences in the way FDA schedules and performs international inspections.

Scheduling. One of the most obvious differences between domestic and international inspections involves the way in which firms are notified of pending inspections. International companies are almost always notified in advance of the FDA visit and firms are generally allowed to negotiate dates that are mutually agreeable to the FDA and the firm. Unlike domestic inspections, where the FDA often does not give advanced notice to the firm being inspected, international inspections are preplanned and typically follow a schedule that is determined in advance of the trip. In some cases, the FDA may even allow firms to propose alternate dates for the FDA to visit their facility.

For logistical reasons, it is almost a necessity for the FDA to conduct international inspections on a scheduled basis where a certain amount of time is allotted for the inspection. This requires that the inspection be conducted and completed within the allotted time period, since there will be several other firms on the itinerary. In addition, logistical considerations make it unrealistic for FDA personnel to travel overseas without a planned itinerary and confirmed reservations for air flights and hotel reservations. It would be counterproductive for the FDA to attempt unannounced inspections at international sites when FDA investigators have no idea of the location of manufacturing sites (frequently in remote or outlying areas). Unannounced inspections may find the plant to be shut down for holidays or maintenance, or English-speaking personnel may not be available. Finally, the site to be inspected may not yet be ready to produce the product that is the subject of the PAI. In certain countries, the FDA must obtain clearance from the Department of State to allow travel by government officials in restricted areas.

There are also legal reasons why FDA international inspections are always planned in advance and firms are notified of the planned schedule. The FDA's authority to perform inspections under sections 704(a)(1)(a) and 704(a)(2)(b) of the FD&C Act does not extend beyond the borders of the United States. Therefore, before scheduling an international inspection, the FDA must seek a company's permission to enter their premises and perform a GMP inspection. Although the FD&C Act does not provide for international inspections, companies that desire to market their products within the United States are effectively required to allow FDA inspections. If a company were to refuse FDA permission to conduct an inspection of an international facility, the FDA would simply prohibit the company from marketing their products in the United States. This would be accomplished through enforcement of the applicable provisions in Chapter VIII of the

FD&C Act. Thus, for these and other reasons, the FDA nearly always provides advanced notice of pending international inspections.

Language Barriers. A common obstacle during FDA international inspection is the language barrier, which results when the FDA personnel are unable to read, write, or communicate in the native language of the firm being inspected. Although a few FDA personnel may be fluent in a foreign language, firms should expect English to be the language used by the FDA personnel. The FDA expects each company to have available personnel who can translate information for the FDA investigator. It is essential for each international company to ensure that personnel are available who can accurately translate documents for the FDA, as well as to translate from English to their native language any relevant information that may be provided by the FDA investigator (e.g., comments, observations, and written reports).

Although the responsible production and quality control personnel in most international facilities are fluent in English, the use of local expressions or colloquialisms may cause translation difficulties. The practical way to overcome communication difficulties is to fully discuss each item and to have questions and answers restated by both parties. Translation accuracy can be improved by having both the requester and recipient rephrase each question several different ways and then having each answer restated by the FDA personnel.

Duration. Typically, international inspections are of shorter duration than domestic inspections. Unlike domestic inspections where the FDA has to collect documentary evidence to support possible litigation, the same burden of proof is not required during international inspections. This allows international inspections to be performed in a shorter period of time compared with domestic inspections. In addition, during domestic inspections, the FDA has almost unlimited freedom to continue the inspection for as long as the investigator deems necessary. In the absence of a predetermined schedule, there is a tendency for inspections to last longer than when there is a target for completion.

When inspecting domestic firms, the FDA has the responsibility over all products manufactured and may extend the inspection to include other products. At foreign facilities, the FDA generally has interest only in products that will be marketed in the United States. For example, in a large facility that markets a single product in the United States, the FDA inspections will cover only the single product.

Finally, most international inspections are completed within the predetermined time frames because failure to do so may interfere with other inspections or international travel schedules that may be difficult to change on short notice. In contrast, during domestic inspections, an FDA inspector may interrupt the inspection (e.g., for holiday, other priority work elsewhere, or to perform extended reviews of documents that have been collected during an inspection). In such cases, the investigator may return to the facility days or weeks later to finish the inspection that was considered to be in-progress. In contrast, international inspections normally follow a predetermined schedule and with rare exceptions (such as finding of serious problems) the inspection will end at the predetermined time.

Frequency of Re-Inspection. FDA re-inspections at international sites are less frequent (i.e., the interval between inspections is longer) compared with the inspection intervals at domestic facilities. As a general rule the FDA would like to follow the same frequency for re-inspection (2-year cycle) for both domestic and international facilities; however, this is not the current practice. The FDA will not approve a product for marketing unless all sites listed in the application have been inspected in the last 2 years. There are a number of reasons to account for this difference, not the least of which is the relative ease with which the FDA can schedule visits to domestic facilities. Such visits at domestic sites may involve little or no direct costs and relatively short periods of time. Conversely, international inspections are limited by budgetary and resource issues. Consequently, it is not uncommon for some international firms that are marketing their products in the United States to have gone without an FDA re-inspection for a period of several years. Another reason for the difference in inspection frequency involves the provisions of the FD&C Act, section 501(h), which contains a statutory requirement for the FDA to inspect each registered facility at least once every 2 years prior to 1998. The statutory requirement did not apply to facilities located outside the United States because they were not required to register with the FDA. The FDA Reform Act of 1997 now requires registration by pharmaceutical manufacturers located in the United States and foreign countries.

2. Pre-Inspection Preparation Techniques Used by the FDA

The FDA's preparation for an inspection is typically the same for domestic and international facilities. The primary difference for international inspections is the option for the FDA investigator to travel to the FDA headquarters offices in Rockville, MD, for the purpose of having pre-inspection briefings. Before departure on an international trip, the FDA inspection teams may be briefed for 2 to 3 days, during which they have the opportunity to meet directly with the staff from various headquarters units and to review original copies of NDAs, Drug Master Files (DMFs), and any records that may have been sent by the company (e.g., pre-inspection summaries). For example, the inspection team may meet with FDA staff from CDER or CBER.

During such meetings, the inspection team discusses strategies with the chemists or microbiologists who have reviewed applications and the compliance staff that have may have been involved in reviewing previous inspection results. In addition, the inspection team will meet with staff from the foreign inspection group within the DEIO. The DEIO office maintains certain copies of the EIRs for all international inspections, and the inspection team has the opportunity to review all previous inspections. During fiscal year 1997 the inspection files for drug manufacturers were transferred from DEIO to CDER. Where significant problems have been detected in the past, the inspection team will copy previous reports and use the information to prepare a strategy for follow-up. The inspection team will also review correspondence between the FDA and the company to be inspected. They will be especially alert for corrective actions that may have been promised, or for responses that reflect incomplete or inappropriate actions from problems that were cited by the FDA during previous inspections. Finally, the inspection team may be coached by FDA reviewers or compliance personnel about areas of concern, priority issues that are to be addressed, or any other guidance as appropriate. For example, if the NDA reviewers have noticed information or data that seem unusual or suspicious, they will identify strategies for investigation during the FDA inspection.

Additional details about FDA pre-inspection preparation techniques were described by Tetzlaff in a three-part series *Validation Issues for New Drug Development*. Planning and preparation techniques that are used by FDA investigators is described in Part II, "Systematic Assessment Strategies" [R. F. Tetzlaff, *Pharmaceutical Technology*, September 1992, October 1992, and January 1993].

B. Preparing for a PAI

Experience has shown that FDA international inspections proceed most smoothly for firms that have experienced prior FDA inspections. International firms with little or no prior FDA experience can do several things to facilitate the FDA inspection. FDA requirements, expectations, and inspection techniques are well known. If personnel fully understand what to expect, there should be few surprises, and companies can avoid many of the serious problems that some international companies have experienced during the past few years. Systematic preparation techniques should be used by international companies that want to maximize the probability of a successful FDA inspection. This section focuses on the following five elements: (1) assigning responsibilities for PAI readiness; (2) determining the PAI schedule; (3) anticipating FDA needs; (4) verifying application integrity; and (5) verifying GMP compliance.

1. Establishing Responsibilities for PAI Readiness

Being ready for a PAI requires effective coordination between every unit or department within the company. Preparing for a PAI can be a project that has definable objectives and responsibilities. PAI readiness is a state that is obtained when each department has conducted the activities needed to assure accuracy of information filed with the FDA and to assure that the firm has achieved GMP compliance. There are a number of ways to assign responsibilities for PAI readiness. One practical approach is for top management to designate one senior person to have the overall authority to assure activities are performed according to the predetermined schedule that is dictated by the planned filing of the NDA/ANDA. The PAI project director is usually a vice president or director-level position within the company. The person often works in the production department or the Quality Assurance/Quality Control unit.

This person should have the authority and power to direct personnel to perform the actions needed to achieve GMP compliance. Since the person will be working across all of the departments within the company, senior management needs to clearly communicate the role and responsibilities of this person during the PAI preparation phase. This may be accomplished by written memos to department heads, interdepartmental meetings, and one-on-one meetings in which senior management clarifies expectations for their staff.

The PAI project director reports directly to senior management (usually at the vice president or president level). This leader has the first-hand knowledge of all aspects of the day-to-day operations of the facility and is skilled at coordinating the activities of multiple departments. The person knows how to facilitate the actions of others to ensure tasks are accomplished in a timely manner. The project director is well versed in FDA expectations and has experience in dealing with FDA inspections. It is expected that the PAI project director will be the main coordinator and company spokesman during the actual PAI inspection.

Although it is not frequently performed, it is desirable for the roles and responsibilities of the PAI project director to be included in a written directive from the senior management to the heads of each unit within the company. A written directive clearly communicates management's expectations and may minimize potential misunderstandings or may eliminate disputes from arising during the project. Clearly defined responsibilities may minimize potential for conflicts that arise between departments when there are conflicting priorities or overlapping responsibilities during the course of PAI preparation.

PAI projects should have a defined management team that is made up of responsible representatives of each major department within the company (e.g., Quality Assurance/Quality Control, Regulatory Affairs, Product or Process Development Units, and Laboratories). Each department should have a primary and secondary representative and an alternate person to serve as a backup if needed. The membership of the PAI readiness team should be posted, and areas of responsibility should be defined in writing. In principle, the responsibilities for PAI readiness in each department are no more than performing normal job functions. However, there are some important distinctions that need to be considered. The most important factor in becoming ready for a PAI is the issue of timing. Production and control activities for each of the various departments need to be conducted according to time frames and milestones that are consistent with the planned filing of the NDA and the subsequent PAI inspection.

The PAI readiness team should meet on a regular basis. The frequency will depend on many factors, but should be often enough to ensure effective communication at key stages of the project. During the early stages, monthly meetings may suffice, but during the final months leading up to the PAI, meetings may need to take place more often.

Minutes of meetings should be circulated to all affected departments and to senior management. Copies of the minutes should be kept in the PAI project file. A primary purpose of such meetings is to judge the progress being made to project milestones. Team members are given the opportunity to discuss problems or difficulties meeting the planned time frames and to consider the need to adjust priorities and work schedules. If unrealistic time frames have been established, the team members can consider making appropriate adjustments.

Another important function of the PAI readiness team is to verify that the organizational responsibilities for their respective units have been defined. The FDA will often given priority attention to reviewing the documents that describe responsibilities of the organizational units that are responsible for GMP compliance. If the PAI readiness team addresses this matter during the early phases of the project, there is a greater likelihood that adequate documentation will be available during the time of the PAI. If the PAI is to cover a newly formed company, then the PAI readiness team may also be responsible for creating such documents.

The PAI readiness team should establish procedures for coordinating PAI activities. This aspect is important for any company that is undergoing a PAI, but is especially critical for international companies. The PAI team must coordinate activities between departments within their own company and must establish effective ways to communicate with the FDA. Ideally, the PAI team should develop a written standard operating procedure (SOP) that defines each step necessary to file applications, establish schedules for the PAI, and other aspects dealing with the FDA. International facilities that have never undergone a PAI may benefit from the experiences of their counterparts in the United States who have been through the PAI process. If practical, international companies should have on their team one or more delegates that have had experience with the PAI process.

The PAI readiness team is made up of senior representatives from each department (e.g., Quality Assurance/Quality Control, Development, and Regulatory Affairs). The members should already have the authority and responsibility for ensuring activities are accomplished according to the predetermined schedule. However, during most projects, conflicting priorities emerge and there is a need to resolve the conflicts in an expeditious manner. The PAI readiness team should develop a simple procedure for identifying such conflicts and to establish procedures to delegate the appropriate tasks and to decide priorities. When necessary, the team members should work together to reach mutually agreeable resolutions to conflicting priorities, and, if necessary, should elevate the issues to senior management to achieve rapid resolution.

The PAI readiness team should identify their key personnel and take steps to assure they will be present during the FDA inspection. They may want to provide training on how to interact with the FDA. Once a firm agrees to a date for the PAI, it needs to inform all key personnel so that they may adjust planned vacations, holidays, or other commitments that may pose conflicts. The PAI readiness team should ensure that there are personnel who are fluent in English to translate questions and answers and to assure that comments and statements made by the FDA are translated for their own employees.

The PAI readiness team will spend considerable time and effort reviewing the documents that have been created during the development project. For new facilities and/or new products, this will require development of documentation systems. Since the PAI readiness team members are usually those who have actually developed the documentation system, these persons will play an important role during PAI. Their familiarity with the records (i.e., identification schemes, filing locations of documents, and retention practices) will permit the team to prepare lists that identify available supporting records and the location of the records for retrieval. Many multinational firms do work at a variety of different sites, and it is important to ensure that records and data are retained at the location(s) where the activities were performed. For example, the FDA expects laboratory data (raw data and original records) to be retained at the site where testing is performed and batch production records to be kept at the plant where batches were formulated; data from testing at contract laboratories would be inspected at the contractor's facility. FDA does not want companies to move records from their original storage locations for the purpose of the FDA inspection. As necessary, the FDA inspection team(s) will go to the facilities where the various activities were performed to inspect the raw data and original records. For example, FDA teams may visit several different countries to inspect the related facilities for a single PAI product.

The PAI readiness team plays an important role in preparing employees for the actual PAI. The team identifies key personnel in each department (managers, supervisors) and provides appropriate orientation. Such orientation identifies their respective roles and responsibilities, and includes training in how to deal with the FDA investigators. These employees are given assignments to perform certain duties within their respective work groups, and advise their direct reports on what to expect and how to act during the PAI.

The PAI readiness team will ensure that the company prepares a development report for the product to be covered by the PAI. Frequently, the PAI team members are those who were directly responsible for preparing the development report and determining its content. In other cases, the PAI readiness team reviews reports that have been prepared by other departments. The PAI readiness team should ensure that the development report is available when the FDA arrives to conduct the PAI.

The ultimate responsibility of the PAI readiness team is to decide what conditions must be satisfied before the facility is considered to be ready for the PAI. Companies that have been unsuccessful in gaining approval from the FDA usually have not accomplished one or more tasks that have been deemed essential by the FDA. For example, a common reason for withholding approval of NDAs is the FDA finding one or more processes that have not been validated, incomplete documentation, and inappropriate or insufficient stability data. The PAI readiness should identify the key elements or criteria that are needed to be "PAI ready."

The criteria may be listed in a simple outline form that is organized by department or quality systems. The listing(s) may include elements that are essential as well as those that are optional (desirable). Examples of essential elements might include the following: (1) formulation and processing steps listed in master formula are the same as those filed in the NDA; (2) every analytical method used in testing of the NDA product has been validated, and each method has an approved test procedure that is supported by the validation protocol (i.e., there are test data and validation reports for each method); and (3) stability data are available from three full-scale commercial batches and at room temperature storage confirms the product meets specifications at all test intervals through 12 months. Optional elements might include the following: (1) the development report has been prepared and signed off by all affected departments; (2) three production scale batches have been produced, and validation protocols have been executed; and (3) all validation reports have been signed off as approved.

2. Determine FDA Schedule

The first step in an international inspection by the FDA is a formal request for permission to conduct the inspection. The FDA request is made by the DEIO by telephone or in writing (letter, FAX, or telex). Because each international inspection trip is normally for a 3- to 4-week period during which up to six facilities may be inspected, the FDA must plan the itineraries well in advance. International companies should promptly reply to FDA requests for scheduling and advise in writing whether the dates are acceptable. FDA notification of the PAI schedule is normally 30 to 60 days in advance of the trip, but may be less. Once the FDA schedules a date for the PAI, this schedule is normally followed unless adjustments are needed due to cancellations by other companies or emergency changes to itineraries. It is a rare occurrence for the FDA to arrive sooner than the planned date, and only occurs if agreed upon by the international firm.

If the inspection dates proposed by the FDA are poorly timed due to facility construction or the inability to manufacture the product, firms should make this known and determine if alternative dates are agreeable to the FDA. Some international companies find it difficult to know how to effectively deal with the FDA or how to determine the schedule for an FDA inspection. Using careful planning techniques, this activity can be relatively simple. The key to success is to understand FDA procedures and to make certain that the FDA is aware of when the firm will be ready for the PAI. Timing is one of the most important factors to consider when scheduling the PAI. Companies do not want the FDA to arrive before they have completed the activities that they and the FDA consider to be essential. Conversely, once the essential activities have been completed, companies do not want FDA to delay the PAI. International companies should communicate with the FDA's DEIO as described in Section II.A.2.

PAI may occur any time after the NDA has been filed. In practice, the FDA expects firms to be ready for a PAI when they file the NDA application. At this time, the CMC section contains the regulatory commitments, and the facility should be in substantial compliance with the GMPs. However, most firms file their NDAs before completing all activities that may be the subject of the FDA inspection.

For international inspections, the FDA will normally contact the company to request a date for scheduling purposes. From this point, it is especially important that international companies communicate effectively with the FDA. It is advisable for companies to have a written SOP that contains appropriate instructions and responsibilities for dealing with FDA contacts. It is beyond the scope of this chapter to describe the content of such procedures. However, emphasis is given to the importance of promptly acknowledging the proposed inspection dates. The SOP should spell out pertinent information about FDA organizations and names and titles of key personnel (including mailing addresses, telephone, and fax numbers). International companies are often requested by the FDA to arrange transportation and lodging for the FDA personnel while they are conducting the PAI. Companies would be well advised to understand the logistic issues and strive to facilitate the FDA visit. International companies need to be aware that the FDA investigators are prohibited from accepting gifts or anything of monetary value. Although international companies may arrange for hotel accommodations, the FDA investigator is required to pay for all costs associated with lodging, meals, and any transportation charges.

3. Anticipate FDA Needs

The 1992 Foreign Inspection Guide listed documents that the FDA would like to have available in advance of the inspection. Although the guide was re-issued in May 1996 in a new format (without listing the documents), international companies may find the 1992 version to be a good source of information about the types of documents that are likely to be reviewed during FDA inspections. A number of documents are commonly requested by the FDA during international inspections, and prudent management will ensure they are available as English summaries. The summaries and facility-related drawings should not contain too much detail. The legends or keys to drawings should use commonly used terms, and color coding is often an effective means of improving the quality of schematic drawings. It is in the companies best interest to make such documents accurate and easy to understand, and to provide the type of information that is useful to the FDA. When these documents are well written, the FDA inspection team is likely to use them as exhibits in the EIR.

Although FDA regulations require that documents submitted to the FDA in filings (e.g., NDAs, ANDAs, and DMFs) must be in English, the FDA expects that raw data and original records that are retained at international sites will be in the native language. The FDA has no expectation that companies maintain documents in English (unless English is the firms native language). However, it will facilitate most FDA inspections if firms prepare a number of summary documents in English. If companies include copies of documents in their DMFs or NDAs, the copies should be certified as accurate translations (e.g., master and batch production records, product specifications, analytical methods, sterilization process documentation, and other narrative descriptions of systems and procedures). Certified copies that have been translated into English should be stamped to reflect that the document is a copy. Although translation copies will not contain the signatures of personnel who signed the originals, they may be signed by the person making the translation to show the translation is an accurate copy. The translated version should be stamped "this translation is for information only and is current as of [date of translation]." This avoids the need to revise the translation every time an SOP is revised.

FDA inspections are predictable in nearly every respect. FDA investigators commonly follow the same general approach, nearly always ask for certain key information, and the majority of the inspections cover the same quality systems. Although each FDA investigator, chemist, or microbiologist may have a particular style, approach, or unique set of priorities, there is a surprising similarity in what is covered during most PAIs.

International companies that fully understand FDA procedures can take certain steps to make sure they have available the information that is most likely to be requested by the FDA. Most international companies anticipate what the FDA will review, and they can take proactive steps to ensure that most of the information is readily available and is in a format that can be reviewed by the FDA team.

By preparing summary documents for key development activities, the firm's personnel will understand what activities have occurred and may be better able to explain the information when requested by the FDA team. The summary documents will serve as an aid during the PAI, and will identify sources of records and supporting data. English translations of key summaries will facilitate discussions with the FDA, but generally firms should avoid moving raw data or original records from one site to another. The FDA expects raw data and original records to be retained at the site where GMP activities were performed.

In anticipation of the PAI, personnel should verify that a development report is available and should review its content. If a development report has not yet been approved, it is advisable for one to be finalized before the PAI. Many FDA investigators use the development report to better understand the activities that were conducted during the early formulation, development, scale-up, and the development of analytical methods. Information from the development report may be used by the company's management to present overviews to the FDA about key development activities at the start of an inspection. If development reports are well written and are reasonably complete (substantive), the FDA investigator may find the summary information to be sufficient for the purposes of the PAI. For example, the FDA may not feel it is necessary to audit raw data, or if raw data are reviewed, the audit begins with a favorable impression. Conversely, if the FDA finds that there is no development report, this may be viewed with reservations and the FDA audit may go into greater depth.

The PAI readiness team should take certain basic steps to ensure that the PAI proceeds as smoothly as possible. Each company should develop a written SOP for hosting FDA inspections, and it should include a section on logistical issues. There are a number of activities that should be accomplished well in advance of the scheduled inspection, including the following:

(1) Reserve a conference room for the FDA that is of suitable size and location (proximity to the facility, records, or laboratories).

(2) The FDA conference room should have reasonable amenities such as a conference table and access to a telephone, photocopier, and clerical assistance if needed.

(3) The company should consider having a "PAI command center" that is in close proximity to the FDA conference room. This room can be used as a private meeting site for the firm's personnel and can be used to retain many of the key documents that will be needed during the PAI. The room should

be locked to allow storage of key documents such as copies of the NDAs, certain GMP records, PAI summaries, etc.

A primary function of the PAI readiness team is to prepare summary documents that will be used, if needed, during the PAI. Preparing English summaries is one of the most effective activities that an international company can do to facilitate the PAI. English summaries are designed to provide useful overviews of key information most likely to be requested by the FDA. The FDA has provided considerable insight into the type of information that it will need during the PAI. The FDA has published a number of documents that describe the information they would like to review in advance of the PAI or during the PAI itself. The following documents contain listings of information that is most likely to be reviewed by the FDA inspection teams: Pre-Approval Inspection Program (CP 7346.832); Post-Approval Inspection Program (CP 7346-843); FDA foreign inspection guides (1992 and 1996); and Inspection Operations Manual (IOM Section 500).

Table 7 lists some examples of the types of summary documents that will facilitate an FDA PAI. Each of the summary documents should be in English, and each may be prepared as overhead transparencies. Management may use the transparencies to provide overviews about each system or area of interest to the FDA. Some of the summaries may be used by the firm's management to provide an overview of company operations at the beginning of the inspection. The remaining summaries are prepared in anticipation of FDA questions for selected systems. In these instances, the summaries are available in case the FDA poses questions and clarification is needed. In the event that the FDA team does not cover any of these areas, then the summaries will not be presented to the FDA.

4. Verify Application Integrity

Since the PAI program was revised in 1990 as a consequence of the generic drug scandal, application integrity has become a major focus during most PAIs. The FDA carefully compares information filed in NDAs, DMFs, annual reports, or other filings against raw data and original records on file at the company being inspected. If significant discrepancies are detected, they may be grounds for recommendations to withhold approvals of NDAs or other regulatory sanctions.

Because of the priority attention that is being given by the FDA to application integrity during international inspections, prudent firms will take steps to ensure that information filed with the FDA is accurate and to verify that appropriate amendments or supplements have been filed to cover any changes made since the original submissions. Firms should establish written SOPs for verifying the accuracy of documents filed with the FDA. International companies that file applications with the FDA should have a U.S. agent make the filings on the behalf of the company. In some cases, the U.S. agent may assume responsibilities

Table 7   Examples of Summaries for Presentations During PAIs

Batch record inventory (listing of batches manufactured) 　Clinical batches 　Stability batches 　Biobatches 　Commercial batches 　Batches distributed in the United 　　States 　Batch release status	Computer systems 　Listing of GMP functions 　Hardware inventory 　Software inventory 　Validation status 　Descriptions of key systems
Bulk pharmaceutical chemicals 　Source (name/address/telephone) 　DMF (Reference/authorization 　　letter) 　Summary of manufacturing 　　processes	Development report 　Prospective reports 　Retrospective reports Documentation system 　SOP for SOPs
Business summaries 　Legal status of company(s) 　Mailing addresses, telephone, FAX, 　　e-mail 　Related divisions or subsidiaries 　U.S. affiliates	Drawings (schematics/floor plans) 　Building layout 　Site plan 　Floor plans/room locations for PAI 　　product(s) 　Equipment placement 　Flow diagrams (personnel, materials, 　　and product) 　Room classifications
Calibration program 　Scope of program 　Scheme for identifying calibration 　　status 　Relevant procedures (SOPs)	DMFs 　Inventory of DMFs 　Contracts/agreements per 314.420 　Summary of vendor audits 　Copies (if available) 　Letters of authorization
Change control system 　Overview of program 　Summaries 　Relevant procedures (SOPs)	Drug product 　Process summaries 　Production history (release status)
Cleaning program overview 　Relevant procedures (SOPs) 　Residue limits 　　Drug product 　　Cleaning agents 　Methods validation 　Cleaning validation 　Validation	Engineering drawings 　As-builts for key facilities and 　　equipment Environmental monitoring 　Relevant procedures (SOPs) 　Limits 　Data summaries

Table 7 (continued)

Equipment inventory	Product listings
Names and descriptions	Listing of all products at site
Identification	Listing of products for U.S.
Equipment listed in NDA/ANDA	Listing of U.S. distributors
Failure investigations	Production facility site plan
Overview of procedures	
Time limits	Responsibilities
	Quality control unit
GMP quality systems listing	Production
	Laboratory
Laboratory overview	Management
Floor plans	
Instrument inventory	Validation program
Methods and procedures	Policies and plans
Analytical record system	Protocols (IQ, QQ, PQ) and reports
Sample receiving and storage	Qualification summaries
Sample accountability	Process validation summaries
	Processes
NDA/ANDA	Product (3-lot validation)
CMC section	
Amendments/supplement inventories	Water systems
	System description
Organizational charts	Schematic drawings
Key personnel (names/titles)	Monitoring limits
Reporting relationships	Data summaries
Chain of command	Validation protocols and reports
Processes	Various Others
Summaries	(as approprite to specific NDA)
Flow diagrams	
Procedures (SOPs)	
Specifications and process parameters	
Validation	

DMF, drug master file; SOP, standard operating procedures; GMP, good manufacturing procedures; PAI, pre-approval inspection; NDA, new drug application; ANDA, abbreviated new drug application; IQ, installation qualification; OQ, operational qualification; PQ, product/process/or performance qualification.

for preparing the CMC sections or the DMF. Errors or discrepancies may go undetected unless companies establish systems for double checking the accuracy of information filed on their behalf by the U.S. agent. FDA investigators are alert for discrepancies during PAIs.

Before a PAI, each firm should perform internal audits to ensure that factually correct, accurate, and complete information is contained in NDAs and ANDAs. An internal audit should be one of the final steps before requesting an FDA inspection under the Pre-Approval Inspection Program (CP7346.832). The application integrity audits (mock FDA inspections) systematically compare information that is contained in applications against raw data and original records. Such audits serve two important purposes. First, they allow the firm a final opportunity to have an independent verification that information in applications is accurate and is supported with raw data. Second, it provides plant personnel with the chance to undergo a simulated FDA-style audit, which provides valuable experience for those having to answer questions and locate supporting documentation. Such audits also provide management with the opportunity to observe how well their key personnel deal with the pressures of an audit and how effectively they communicate. Management may use this experience to decide the person's role during the scheduled FDA inspection and may find it necessary to provide additional training or instructions on how to be more effective during audit situations.

5. Verify GMP Compliance

FDA expectations for GMP compliance are the same for domestic and international companies. Products marketed within the United States must conform to the GMP regulations (21 CFR Part 211), and where applicable, they must meet the requirements of the United States Pharmacopeia (USP). International companies that produce products for both the United States and other international markets may need to establish dual procedures, testing methods, and specifications or release limits to ensure they conform with FDA requirements as well as those of local regulatory authorities. When companies have dual requirements, it is imperative that employees be given training in both. Steps should be taken to ensure that employees work to the highest standard and that they follow the correct procedures, test methods, and release specifications that are applicable to batches intended for the U.S. market.

For the same reasons described for application integrity audits, it is advisable to perform internal GMP audits before the PAI. Such audits may focus on product development, scale-up to full-size production batches, qualification of equipment and utilities, validation of processes and laboratory methods, batch records and SOPs, and any other area. International companies have been receiving priority attention by the FDA in recent years, and during FY 1995, 42% of the international inspections resulted in recommendations to withhold approval of NDAs or ANDAs. In Section IV, some examples of common FDA findings in international facilities are reviewed.

C. Hosting International PAIs

Although hosting FDA inspections is generally the same for domestic and international facilities, there are certain inherent differences due to language barriers and the challenges that are posed when personnel try to keep abreast of FDA requirements and expectations from remote international sites. While FDA documents (e.g., guidelines, inspection guides, and various inspection programs) are readily available to everyone, personnel in international facilities face a greater challenge than their U.S. colleagues. Companies that do not have U.S. facilities frequently lack experience in dealing with the FDA during inspections, and they may face difficulties during the inspection if key personnel are not fully knowledgeable about the GMP regulations and FDA requirements inspection practices.

Probably the largest obstacle to most international inspections is the language barrier. Key liaison personnel are needed to ensure effective communications between the FDA and personnel at the facility being inspected. In instances where management is not fluent in English, then translators will be necessary to expedite the inspection and to ensure accurate information is provided. FDA personnel may use expressions or colloquialisms that are unfamiliar to international personnel, which makes translations difficult and may lead to misunderstandings. If personnel are uncertain about terms and acronyms used by the FDA, they are advised to ask for clarification before answering questions or providing information. Some companies have found it helpful to have U.S. representatives from their parent organization accompany the FDA investigator during international PAIs. Having a U.S. representative present may be especially beneficial when NDAs or DMFs have been prepared or filed by a U.S. agent or the firms corporate offices located in the United States. These representatives may provide clarification and interpretation about information contained in filings and can assist local management in understanding FDA inspection practices and regulatory requirements.

Personnel at foreign companies are usually good about providing common courtesies to the FDA inspection team. Such courtesies include offering a work area that afford some privacy if needed by a team, a conference room for conducting the inspection that includes, if needed, a photocopier, telephone, and fax machine. It is appropriate to provide the FDA with refreshments such as coffee, tea, etc., but the FDA considers it to be inappropriate to accept meals or anything of monetary value. FDA personnel will want to pay for their own meals (even at a company cafeteria). Companies that provide meals in their cafeteria or at a local restaurant should allow the FDA team members to contribute their share of the costs. They should honor the FDA personnel's requests to pay for their meals, and should allow payment in as discreet manner as practical. It is inadvisable for management to insist on paying or to question the FDA team members why they are insisting to pay. Some companies normally provide international visitors with small gifts as tokens of appreciation, but this custom should be avoided for members of an FDA inspection team.

Hosting an FDA inspection team during an international PAI requires careful planning and coordination to ensure that all key personnel understand their duties and responsibilities during the period the FDA inspection team is present. International companies almost always are made aware of the FDA inspection schedule and know exactly when the inspection team will arrive. This permits senior management to adjust their schedules to ensure they are present when the FDA arrives. The key liaison person should brief the FDA team, and it is often effective to introduce the team to the senior-most management official at the local site. After these preliminary introductions, it is customary to move to the conference room that has been set aside for the FDA inspection. At this point, it is advisable for the company to assemble a small group of the key managers who are expected to be available to assist during the PAI. These personnel should be introduced and their area of their area of responsibility explained.

At the onset, the lead FDA investigator will normally explain the purpose of the inspection, the expected duration of the visit, and will make known any special requests for records or other needs. At this point, companies should feel free to pose questions to the inspection team to better understand the objective and scope of the inspection, so that management can assure that key personnel are available to meet the needs of the FDA inspection team. For example, it would be appropriate to ask which areas of the facility are to be explained by the FDA during the course of the inspection so that key personnel can be scheduled to be available when needed. Although the FDA may not know exactly which areas are to be visited or when, they will normally advise management of the scope and will indicate whether the visit will extend to the production areas, laboratories, research facilities, or other specific departments within the facility.

Most FDA investigators prepare an inspection outline that they will use to guide the inspection. There is certain key information that will nearly always be requested by the inspection team. International companies should offer to provide a short presentation to the FDA inspection team. This presentation should use the English summaries that had been previously prepared (described in Section III.B.3). During this initial presentation, management should offer to provide an overview of the company, including the organizational structure, description of the manufacturing sites, laboratories, and other areas that are pertinent to the PAI. The presentation should describe the types of products manufactured, an area or site map should be presented, and floor plans and plant layout diagrams should be available in case the investigators have questions about where the various activities are performed.

The duration of this initial presentation should be relatively short (approximately 15 to 30 minutes), but management should observe FDA's reaction to this presentation. If the inspection team seems interested and is asking a lot of questions, then the presentation may be extended for a longer period. Management should judge the effectiveness of the presentation, and if the inspection team seems disinterested or anxious to proceed with their inspection, then the presentation should be terminated. Before proceeding to the plant inspection, management should provide the FDA team with an overview of normal company procedures. For example, they should explain the normal business hours, company safety policies and procedures, policies with respect to being escorted in the facility, and any restrictions to controlled areas of the facility. Information should be provided about suitable attire and any security issues such as access to controlled areas or confidential information.

During the initial presentation, management should advise the FDA inspection team that they are interested in being made aware of any findings during the inspection. Management should ask the FDA inspection team if they would be willing to have a short daily discussion (approximately 15 minutes) during which the company is given the opportunity to discuss observations made by the inspection team. It may even be possible to agree to a time schedule each afternoon for such discussion. The purpose of these discussions is to have the FDA inspection team present any areas of concern or problems that may have been noted during the day's visit. During these discussions, management should be careful to solicit from the FDA any observed problems or areas that may be of concern but not yet resolved by the inspection team. These meetings are of considerable advantage to both the inspection team and management of the company. The FDA inspection team will use the meetings to resolve any misunderstandings, and it provides management with the opportunity to learn what areas are of concern to the FDA. Based on these stated concerns, management can reevaluate whether all relevant information has been presented to the inspection team and if not, personnel can assemble all relevant information as appropriate.

Companies should designate a principle person to serve as the liaison for the FDA inspection who will accompany the FDA at all times. During international inspections, the liaison person is frequently someone who has a good command of the English language and is familiar with all aspects of the company's operations. The liaison person should have the authority to obtain the necessary personnel and information that may be requested by the FDA. However, this person should delegate the task of obtaining the various information to other persons so that the liaison can be present at all times. If the FDA inspection includes a team of two or more FDA personnel, it will be necessary to designate multiple personnel to serve as the liaison for each team member. It is not uncommon for FDA team members to divide into two or more groups and operate independently in separate areas of the facilities.

International companies are advised to designate one or more persons to take notes during the course of the FDA inspection. The person taking notes should not be the person serving in the liaison capacity. The person taking notes should maintain a record of the questions that were asked and the answers that were given to each question. At the end of each day, a written transcript summarizing the activities of each day should be prepared. This record need not be an exact transcription of every detail, but should reflect the questions asked by the FDA, the answers provided (and by whom), and any significant observations or recommendations made by the FDA personnel. The record should also note any misunderstanding or potential disagreements that may have become apparent. Having a permanent record of the progress of the FDA inspection may be valuable at later stages, such as when attempting to prepare a response to an FDA 483 observation or to understand the reasons behind FDA objections. During FDA team inspections, it is advisable to have separate persons taking notes whenever the FDA team divides into groups.

Most FDA inspections devote considerable time reviewing batch production and control records. During international inspections, it is customary for the FDA to request documents that are retrieved by company personnel and brought to the FDA conference room. In most cases, the FDA investigators will allow management to retrieve documents and bring them to the FDA personnel. However, in some cases, the inspection team may request to observe the document filing systems or to observe the storage locations for the original records. When this happens, personnel should be prepared to deal with the request. The company should retain duplicate photocopies of documents that have been provided to the inspection team, and they should be filed with the daily inspection summary.

International companies commonly are unsure of the FDA position regarding photographs during FDA inspections. The FDA typically photographs violative conditions or observed conditions. Each firm should establish a written procedure that defines its position regarding whether it will allow FDA to take photographs. Procedures should be reviewed by the company's legal counsel. For domestic companies, refusal to permit photographs may result in the FDA obtaining an inspection warrant, but this option is not available during international inspections. When deciding whether to allow photographs, international companies should take into account the potential impact that a refusal may have on the FDA inspection team. If met with a refusal, the inspection team would not take photographs during an international inspection. However, the team may use other options, such as taking samples, or making copies of additional records to support the observations.

International companies may wish to consider other alternatives. It may be preferable to explain to the FDA team that the company is not refusing to allow photographs to be taken, but is concerned with maintaining proprietary or confidential trade secret information. The company could request that before allowing photographs to be taken, it would like the opportunity to determine if any confidential information may be compromised by the photographs. Most FDA investigators would view this as reasonable and would probably agree to such a request. In some cases, it would not be advisable to carry an FDA camera into a controlled environment. The company may wish to offer to use their own equipment, which can be sanitized or disinfected before being taken into controlled environments, and to provide the FDA personnel with the photographs that are requested. If the FDA inspection team takes photographs during an inspection, the company is advised to have their own photographer take duplicate pictures of the same areas. After the FDA inspection, international companies should request from the FDA copies of the photographs that were taken by the inspection team. The FDA policy is to provide such copies if the international companies pay the commercial fees for developing the film.

Firms should establish written SOPs that describe responsibilities and activities that are to be followed by their personnel during an FDA inspection. Training should be provided to each person who is intended to participate in the FDA inspection to ensure that they understand and follow established procedures. The following are some practical training issues to be considered; prudent management will consider additional factors.

The procedures should clearly establish practical details such as who will accompany the visitors, what information may be expected to be requested, what information may not be provided (such as financial data), procedures to be followed if problems develop, etc. Firms desire FDA inspections to proceed with minimum delays and do not want confrontational situations to develop. One practical way to avoid confrontations is to ensure that the firm's personnel fully understand FDA inspection objectives and know what information and records to which the FDA are entitled access. If firms establish effective procedures for dealing with requests in a courteous and professional manner, disagreements and problems may be largely eliminated.

The procedure should describe the FDA's authority for conducting inspections and its access to records. Under section 704 of the FD&C Act, the FDA is given authority to review all records that have a bearing on conformance with cGMPs. FDA investigators performing international inspections would expect to see the same type of records as they would for domestic inspections (although there are certain legal differences that are not discussed in this chapter). FDA authority to examine records does not extend to financial data, personnel data (except GMP training records), sales data, or research data (except in support of an application). International companies should designate a key management person to be responsible for reviewing FDA requests for access to records. If FDA requests seem to be outside the scope of section 704, then the matter should be referred to the key person for resolution. Before an international company refuses to provide access to particular records, it is advisable to have an open discussion with the inspection team concerning their right to access to these documents. The FDA inspection team should be able to defend their request for access to certain records.

One of the most important aspects of hosting an FDA inspection is dealing with deficiencies or problems that have been detected by the inspection team. International companies should strive to understand the FDA investigator's objections. If at all possible, the company should attempt to make corrections while the inspection is still in progress. The corrective actions taken in response to an FDA observation should be pointed out to the FDA during the daily discussions and again during the discussion of the FDA-483. FDA personnel are expected to report corrective actions in the EIR. When it is not possible to complete the corrective actions before the FDA leaves the premises, it is in the firm's best interest to report steps that have already been taken toward initiating a corrective action plan. In addition, the FDA is concerned about the steps taken to prevent recurrence of such problems and the evaluations made to determine if the objectionable conditions may apply to other areas of the facility, as well as the steps taken by the company to determine the cause of specific objections found by the FDA. International companies are cautioned against reporting that a particular observation has been corrected when the cause of the problem has not been addressed. During FDA follow-up inspections, most FDA investigators will look for new areas of the facility where the same or similar problems may exist (even though the specific items listed on the previous FDA-483 may have been corrected).

International companies that do not have prior experience with FDA inspections may fail to fully appreciate the importance of application integrity issues to the FDA inspection team. FDA team members are especially alert for any data that seem suspicious or may otherwise suggest conditions or practices other than described in the applications made to the FDA. Some FDA investigators have found that personnel may have falsified records, changed procedures or practices contrary to applications, or they may have been given false information by employees during FDA inspections. As a consequence, FDA investigators are trained to be alert for such signals or clues as: (1) answers that seem evasive or inconsistent; (2) unexpected behavior (such as body language or eye contact); or (3) inconsistent answers between employees. International companies should provide training to the personnel that are likely to be involved with the FDA inspection so that they understand why FDA inspections may focus on application integrity issues.

International companies frequently find it desirable to have the FDA inspection team join them for dinner to provide the opportunity for plant personnel to get to know the inspection members and to discuss FDA matters. This is considered to be appropriate as long as the FDA team members are allowed to pay for their own meals. International companies may want to discuss this issue with the inspection team and consent to their preferences. While dinner meetings are entirely appropriate, companies should avoid activities that would be viewed as entertainment or social functions. While the companies may provide common courtesies, they should not "roll out the red carpet," or place the inspection team in a difficult position.

D. Responding to FDA Observations

When the FDA completes its inspection, the final action is to have an exit discussion with management to discuss the inspection findings. If the FDA team has detected GMP deviations or other objectionable conditions, they will leave with the company a written list of observations (FDA-483), and will provide management with the opportunity to discuss the FDA findings. The purpose of the FDA-483 is to list objectionable conditions and practices found by the FDA investigator; it is not intended to report any favorable or acceptable conditions that may have been observed during the inspection. The FD&C Act [Section 704(b)] requires the FDA personnel to "provide written descriptions of any [conditions or practices which] in his judgment indicate any . . . drug . . . consists in whole or part of any filthy, putrid, or decomposed substance, or (2) has been prepared, packed or held under insanitary conditions whereby it may have been contaminated with filth, or whereby it may have been rendered injurious to health."

The observations listed on the FDA-483 represent conditions that the FDA team believes to be objectionable or unacceptable, but this is not necessarily the FDA's final word on the matter. Each FDA-483 is subjected to further review by FDA management in the field offices and/or at headquarters units to determine the validity and significance of each item. It is imperative that personnel completely understand the reason(s) that FDA considers a condition or practice to be objectionable before the inspection team departs.

International companies that have had daily discussions with the FDA should not be surprised by the observations that are listed on the FDA-483. In fact, they should anticipate most of the objections and be prepared to discuss each item. Each item should be read out loud so that key personnel can understand the content. If necessary, a representative of the international facility may translate each item individually to ensure that every person who is present clearly understands each observation.

Management is encouraged to verbally respond to the inspection findings during the discussion of the FDA-483. Each item should be discussed individually, and the company personnel should provide additional explanations where appropriate, and should state their intentions for items where they have made or intend to make improvements. When companies have initiated corrective actions, it is imperative that the FDA be informed of the actions taken (especially corrections that have already been completed). The company should request that the FDA team report in their EIR that the corrections that have been accomplished. If the FDA has had the opportunity to verify the corrections, it would be appropriate to ask them to comment on the adequacy of the actions taken by the company (i.e., were they satisfied with the corrective actions or should the firm consider further actions?).

Where practical, the firm may present the FDA team with copies of documents that show corrections such as revised SOPs, change control records for facility improvements, training documentation, and results of analytical testing. Where the firm may need some time to decide appropriate corrective actions, it is advisable to inform the FDA team that a written response will be provided within a reasonable period (ideally within 2 weeks). Since commitments that are made by management will be reported in the EIR, it is important for them to be realistic. For example, making promises that are based on unrealistic timetables or that may be conditional on factors that are outside the firms direct control (such as capital expenditures that may have unexpected delays) should be avoided. If the FDA finds during follow-up inspections that commitments have gone unfulfilled, this will lead to credibility problems with the FDA and may result in regulatory actions.

The FDA encourages an open discussion of each item listed on the FDA-483, and the FDA team should be able to defend its observations. If management believes an item listed on the FDA-483 is incorrect or does not accurately reflect the true conditions found by the FDA investigator, this should be discussed in sufficient detail until the issue can be resolved to mutual satisfaction. If the observation is an error due to misunderstandings, it is essential that there be full discussions to ensure that the FDA has accurate and complete information. If the FDA has all of the relevant information and facts, but the FDA team has reached the conclusion that the firms practices or conditions are unacceptable, then the FDA-483 observation will remain. However, if new or different information is provided that changes their conclusions about the listed objection, then the item may be deleted or revised during the exit discussion. To revise or delete an item, the FDA team may make a hand written annotation or may strike the item by simply drawing a line through the observation. Alternatively, the FDA may rewrite a page of the FDA-483 to remove the item that was found to be incorrect.

When management disagrees with an observation that the FDA team declines to delete or revise, the firm should: (1) identify what data and information were used by the FDA as the basis for their observations; (2) verify that the company has the same information and data that were used by the FDA to make their point; (3) if the firm believes the FDA has not considered certain information or data that are relevant, then provide additional records or explanations; (4) if the company believes the FDA has the correct information and data but have reached a conclusion that is invalid, then try to understand the logic or rationale used by the FDA; (5) ask the FDA to explain the basis or reason why they believe the condition or practice is objectionable (e.g., is the observation based on their opinions or are there published documents that define the FDA position on the particular matter [such as FDA regulations, policies, guidelines, or published papers in scientific journals]); (6) when all attempts have failed to convince the FDA to revise its position, the company should clearly restate their position and the reasons and request that the FDA team include in their EIR report that the company does not believe the FDA observation is valid and their basis for disagreement (if possible, the FDA team should be provided with a written statement before they leave the premises); and (7) after the FDA inspection prepare a response that states the firm's disagreement and the reasons.

When the FDA team has not found objectionable conditions, they will terminate the inspection (an FDA-483 will not be issued). In such cases, the company will not receive anything in writing from the FDA team, but it is important for the company to request a final exit discussion meeting where management discusses the results of the inspection with the FDA personnel. Management should ask the FDA team to confirm that they have not found any objectionable conditions, and to determine whether anything was found that may result in a recommendation to withhold approval of an NDA/ANDA or other filings. An appropriate question to ask the FDA investigator is "Do you plan to recommend approval of the NDA for [name product]?"

For international inspections, the FDA team normally prepares its written EIR after the team returns to the United States. Prudent management will determine when the FDA is expected to return to the United States and the expected timetable for completing the EIR. The firm should make sure that its written response to any FDA-483 observations arrives at the FDA office before the EIR is completed. Timing is important because FDA management decisions will take into account the firm's response. Ideally, the response should be submitted within about 2 weeks of the issuance of the FDA-483, but the time may be more or less as dictated by the significance of the findings. If the firm's written response is delivered to the DEIO office by the time the EIR is being reviewed, then the

FDA's recommendations will be based on the EIR and the company's response. Thus, it is in the company's best interest to respond in a timely and thoughtful manner.

Original FDA-483 responses and support documentation should be sent to Mr. Joseph Famulare, Director, Division of Manufacturing and Product Quality (HFD-320), Metro Park North (MPN-1), 7520 Standish Place, Rockville, MD 20855.

Additional copies of the firm's response to the FDA-483 should be forwarded to the following FDA offices to ensure that key FDA personnel receive the information directly from the company. Although it might seem unnecessary to send multiple copies to so many locations, it is in the firm's best interest to send responses to FDA-483s to: (1) Division of Emergency and Investigational Operations (DEIO) (HFC-133); (2) CDER, Office of Compliance, Foreign Inspection Team (HFD-322); and (3) to each member of the inspection team. See Tables 2 and 4 for addresses and telephone numbers.

Firms should deliver a copy of their written responses to each FDA inspection team member (FAX a copy and send another copy by overnight delivery service to confirm receipt). Send the response to the mailing addresses that were provided by the team during the inspection. If copies of the firm's FDA-483 response reach the FDA inspection team before they complete the EIR, they will likely consider the responses. If persuasive information is provided, they may even modify their positions on particular issues before the EIR is completed. If the team members have already received the response directly from the company, they will be able to provide a timely evaluation of the adequacy of the response when requested by the DEIO or CDER Compliance.

The format of a written response may vary depending on the circumstances, but at a minimum, it will describe management's commitment to achieve corrections and it will provide a detailed response to every cited item. Ideally, the written response will duplicate in its entirety each FDA-483 observation followed by the firm's position for each item. The response should clearly and completely reflect management's intentions to correct any items and to present planned timetables for corrective measures.

FDA officials who decide the outcome of PAI are influenced by the timeliness and appropriateness of responses to the FDA-483. FDA officials will likely react negatively when companies fail to respond to an FDA-483 or if the statements lack substantive commitments on the part of management to achieve corrections. The response should include specific action regarding each item with concise statements that are direct and to the point. Responses that are too lengthy or contain excessive irrelevant information may be set aside or reviewed in a cursory manner. The FDA does not want to hear excuses or a repeat of the same points that may have already been rejected during the inspection. However, a simple list of promised actions with no supportive documentation is not convincing and may not be well received by the FDA.

The FDA considers the ideal response to be one that clearly states what action is being taken to correct the situation and the specific actions that have been taken to prevent similar occurrences in the future (or in other systems). The FDA looks for statements that confirm that the cited deficiencies have been eliminated, and will be most comfortable when the response is accompanied by supporting documentation that allows the FDA reviewers to independently verify the corrective actions. Examples of appropriate supporting documents that may be attached to written responses include but are not limited to the following: (1) copies of revised documents such as SOPs or production records; (2) summaries of qualification or validation studies that have been completed since the inspection; (3) photographs of facility modifications or newly installed equipment; (4) copies of invoices or purchase orders for new equipment that has been ordered or installed; (5) summaries showing results of testing performed since the inspection; and (6) corrective action plans with timetables for completion.

When the FDA has cited numerous observations or if findings are considered to be especially significant, it is prudent to develop a corrective action plan that establishes responsibilities and time frames for completion. Senior management should commit to ensuring the corrective action plan will be implemented and completed as promised to the FDA.

Once the lead investigator or analyst completes the EIR, it is forwarded to the local FDA district compliance office that makes a recommendation to approve or withhold approval of the NDA or ANDA. The district recommendation is forwarded to the FDA headquarters unit that is responsible for the application approval (such as CDER or CBER). Unfortunately, the FDA does not have a specific time frame for making their final decision, and the decision could be made as soon as the inspection is completed or not until some months later.

IV. FDA INTERNATIONAL ENFORCEMENT PRACTICES

The FDA requires drugs (including BPCs and finished pharmaceuticals) that are distributed within the United States to be manufactured in facilities that comply with cGMPs. Drugs made under conditions that do not conform to cGMPs are deemed by the FDA to be adulterated within the meaning of Section 501(a)(2)(B) of the FD&C Act. Because the FD&C Act makes no distinction between bulk drug substances and finished pharmaceuticals, the failure of either to comply with cGMPs will be deemed by the FDA to be in nonconformance with the requirements of the Act.

When the FDA detects significant GMP deviations or they find application integrity issues at international facilities, there can be adverse consequences. While the regulatory options that are available to the FDA for international sites are similar to those imposed for domestic companies, there are certain differences that deserve discussion.

After an international inspection there is an administrative review of the documents that have been prepared by the FDA inspection team (FDA-483 and EIR). FDA personnel will evaluate the reported findings and consider the statements made in the firm's response to the FDA-483. Before FY 1997, the administrative review of international inspection reports had been handled by the ITOB office in Rockville, MD (see Section III.B.2) but as a consequence of a recent reorganization, this function has been delegated to the FDA field office where the lead investigator or analyst resides (see Section II.C). The current practice is for the local district management to review the EIR and to make an endorsement using the same procedures and time frames as for domestic inspections. The procedures are described in the FDA Field Management Directive No. 86 (FMD-86). The original EIR and supporting exhibits and the endorsement are forwarded to CDER Office of Compliance (HFD-300) and a copy is sent to the DEIO. The CDER Office of Compliance, Division of Manufacturing and Product Quality Control Foreign Inspection Team (HFD-322) reviews the information submitted by the field office and decides whether to concur with in the field recommendation or an alternative action.

If the international inspection of facilities or systems covered products that have already been marketed within the United States, the Office of Compliance may initiate one or more of the regulatory sanctions that are described in the following sections. Four primary enforcement options are used by the FDA for products that have been produced in international countries and intended for distribution in the United States: (1) withhold approval of pending application or withdraw an approved application; (2) issue a warning letter; (3) invoke Automatic Import Detention; and (4) apply the Application Integrity Policy (AIP) program.

A. Withhold Approval of NDA/ANDA Applications

For international inspections, this is the simplest and most common regulatory option that is used by the FDA when the conditions at the drug manufacturer were found to be in noncompliance with cGMPs (or if application integrity was found to be compromised). Following review the Foreign Inspection Team will forward its recommendation to the Application Evaluation Staff (HFD-324) to withhold approval of the pending application (NDA), and if there is concurrence with the recommendation, the FDA will issue to the company a letter that states the reason(s) why the FDA is not approving the application. If the sponsor receives a letter, it is vital for the firm to fully understand the reasons and to communicate with the FDA their intentions to correct the problems that prevent the agency from granting approval.

In recent years, FDA international inspections have resulted in a relatively high percentage of recommendations to withhold approval of NDAs/ANDAs. For example, for FY 1995, 42% of the international inspections (96 of 230 inspections) resulted in the FDA field offices recommending withholding approval of the application. In FY 1996, 26% of the international inspections resulted in field recommendations to withhold approval. In many instances, firms were eventually able to gain approvals after making corrections and/or re-inspections by the FDA verified that corrective actions were adequate.

B. FDA Warning Letters

The FDA defines a warning letter as "a written communication from the FDA notifying an individual or firm that the agency considers one or more products, practices, processes, or other activities to be in violation of the Federal FD&C Act, or other acts, and that failure of the responsible party to take appropriate and prompt action to correct and prevent any future repeat of the violation, may result in administrative and/or regulatory enforcement action without further notice." A warning letter is intended to reinforce the seriousness of deficiencies found during the inspection and to establish an official prior warning in the event that the FDA decides to proceed with regulatory sanctions. The decision to issue a warning letter is reached after review of the FDA-483, EIR, and the firm's response(s).

Warning letters are issued to senior management, advising them that the inspection findings represent violations of the law and usually listing examples of the more serious findings. The warning letter will also state regulatory actions that may have already been initiated and/or those that are contemplated by the FDA if the firm does not bring their operations into compliance with GMPs. For example, warning letters that are issued after a PAI will often state that the FDA will withhold approval of the pending application (or supplements) until the FDA confirms that adequate corrections have been made. The warning letter may restate some of items that were listed on the FDA-483, and also may cite GMP deviations that were not listed on the FDA-483. Warning letters are used to establish "prior warning" as a basis for future regulatory action. Warning letters may be issued even if the firm has responded to the FDA-483.

Companies that receive a warning letter should give it immediate attention and provide a timely response to the FDA. The response should be delivered to the FDA within 15 working days. Prudent management will make certain that the response is timely and that it adequately addresses all FDA concerns. The response to a warning letter should state corrections already accomplished, actions that have been initiated but are not yet completed (with realistic timetables for completion), and management's commitment to ensure that corrective actions will extend to all operations at the firm. Especially important to the FDA are the actions taken to prevent recurrence of the observed problems and the steps to insure that similar conditions do not exist in the areas that were not specifically covered by the FDA.

Warning letter responses should be concise and should address each point that is cited in the letter. The response should include copies of supporting documentation showing that corrections were substantive. The responses should contain estimates for the time needed to complete corrective actions for items that cannot be immediately corrected.

FDA warning letters normally provide the name of the FDA contact who is responsible for coordinating the FDA follow-up, including scheduling a re-inspection. International companies that receive warning letters should coordinate with FDA officials to ensure re-inspections are scheduled at an appropriate time. Prudent management will keep the FDA well advised of the progress being made to correct the GMP deviations and will advise the FDA of their desires for scheduling the re-inspection. The timing for re-inspection is decided by the FDA, but the company can influence the schedule by keeping the FDA informed about its progress in achieving corrections and/or by notifying the FDA when the firm is ready for the re-inspection. For example, the timing for a re-inspection will depend on a number of factors, including: (1) whether the company has responded to the warning letter; (2) the adequacy of their response; and (3) whether the firm is currently marketing their products within the United States.

The FDA may schedule a follow-up inspection relatively soon after a warning letter if the GMP deviations have a potential impact on products that are being marketed in the United States. If the violative conditions at an international facility involve operations that are not associated with products for the U.S. market (such as a new product that has not yet been distributed in the United States), then the FDA may delay the re-inspection until the firm notifies the FDA that they are ready.

The FDA will normally try to accommodate reasonable requests for re-inspection dates if the international company provides ample notice as to when they will be ready. However, schedules will be subject to availability of personnel, travel funds, and other uncertainties of planning international travel. International companies that request re-inspection after receipt of a warning letter should have taken precautions to ensure that they have corrected the violative conditions. Premature requests for re-inspection may have serious consequences when the FDA finds the violations have not been adequately addressed (or if they find similar deviations in other areas that were not covered by the FDA during the initial inspection). The FDA nearly always considers that their inspections have been relatively limited in scope, and will expect the firm to have addressed the cause(s) of problems detected by the FDA. Follow-up inspections will almost always expand coverage to areas that were not covered during the initial audit. If the FDA finds more GMP deviations, they will consider these to be evidence of continuing noncompliance. International companies should give careful attention to this issue and make certain that corrective actions have extended to all areas of their facility.

If FDA inspections find that the promised corrections were not accomplished, the firm's credibility with the FDA will be damaged and there will be further delays in the approval of the application. If corrections have not been effective and the firm is marketing their products in the United States, the FDA may decide to initiate regulatory sanctions against the international company (such as import detention).

C. Import Detention

This regulatory option is used by the FDA to prevent products that are considered to be adulterated from being imported into the United States. It is an administrative procedure that has been in use since 1974 that permits the U.S. government to refuse products that are offered for entry into the United States. The authority for Import Detention in Section 801(a)(3) of the Act that permits the U.S. government to refuse to allow admission of adulterated drugs into the country, including products that have been manufactured in nonconformance with GMPs or where the FDA finds reasons to suspect the integrity of data submitted to the Agency. Import Detention effectively enjoins a firm from marketing its products in the United States by imposing administrative action against each offered entry. Import Detention does not have an impact on batches of drug products that may have already been introduced into the U.S. market. Once shipments have already entered the United States, the FDA could invoke other sanctions to remove adulterated products from the marketplace, including voluntary recall or seizure.

The FDA will take steps to place products on Import Detention when the Agency considers the GMP deviations to be egregious or when the FDA finds corrections have not been accomplished in a timely fashion. For example, Import Detention may occur if the FDA were to find evidence of cross-contamination, if re-inspection(s) disclosed continuing evidence of noncompliance, or if promised corrections were not achieved. When a firm's products are placed on Import Detention, the products are refused entry into the United States until the FDA inspection(s) confirms that appropriate corrections have been accomplished. The FDA can initiate import detention actions relatively quickly (e.g., a few days or even hours). For example, approximately 3 days after an FDA inspection, the Agency initiated an Import Detention against a firm that refused to disclose to the FDA the location where products were being manufactured. Since Import Detention is an administrative sanction, it can be lifted at the FDA's discretion once the Agency is satisfied that objectionable conditions have been eliminated (i.e., verified by a follow-up inspection at the international firm to confirm corrections).

D. Application Integrity Policy

The Application Integrity Policy (AIP) is a formal administrative program that the FDA uses to deal with fraud, scientific misconduct, or other instances where wrongful acts have been committed or are suspected. The AIP, introduced in 1990 as consequence of the generic drug scandal, was formerly called the "fraud policy." Typically, during PAIs, the FDA will compare data from an application with the raw data from original records at the firm being inspected. The AIP is invoked when the integrity of data or information in applications filed with the FDA has been compromised or questioned. Examples of actions that may prompt investigations include submission of false or fraudulent data, making untrue statements to FDA officials, offering illegal gratuities, and other actions that subvert the integrity of an application.

Since the AIP program was introduced in 1990, a number of firms have been placed on the program. The majority of the AIP actions to date have involved domestic firms, but the AIP has been applied to at least one international company. Once the AIP is initiated against a company, the company is required to initiate investigations to assess the validity of information and data in support of applications. While validity assessments are in progress, the FDA will generally suspend review of pending applications until integrity questions have been resolved. The primary enforcement options that are available to the FDA under the AIP program are as follows:

(1) *Withhold approval of applications*: Pending applications will generally not be reviewed until the FDA completes its validity assessment and

has assurances that questions about data integrity have been resolved. When the company is unable to resolve integrity issues to the FDA's satisfaction, the Agency may refuse to approve applications that are pending or may revoke the approval of applications that have been previously approved.

(2) *Recalls*: The FDA may request firms to voluntarily remove from the market products for which the integrity of supporting data may have been compromised.

(3) *Civil and criminal penalties*: Civil and criminal penalties may be imposed on firms or individuals that have been found to have committed wrongful acts and/or where inaccurate or fraudulent data have been filed in an application. Seizures are administrative actions that may be used by the FDA to prevent drug products from being distributed in interstate commerce. Seizures may be invoked against new drugs for which the applications have been found to contain data that are false or misleading. The FDA may file criminal charges against individuals who are suspected of having committed acts that are in violation of the FD&C Act or other statutes. The FDA has a special unit, Office of Criminal Investigations (OCI), that investigates instances of suspected criminal activities. To date, the authors are aware of only one foreign firm being placed under the AIP. This occurred because the "firm submitted false or misleading information in applications filed with [the] agency" [*FDA Week*, February 28, 1997].

V. SUMMARY

This chapter provided a brief overview of the FDA's international inspection program. Management responsible for handling FDA PAI at international sites need to fully understand the current structure of the FDA, the operations of the FDA's foreign inspection staff, and the applicable FDA requirements and expectations, and they must remain mindful of the consequences of failing to have an acceptable PAI. Practical techniques that may be used to prepare for a PAI inspection were presented. The effectiveness of the techniques used to prepare for the inspection will determine to a large degree whether a firm will have a successful outcome.

Management responsible for facilities located in foreign countries must realize that GMP compliance is not the only factor that determines success. To be certain that the firm is ready for the FDA, it is vital for the firm to ensure readiness of the facility and its staff, provide clear and timely presentations of requested information, ensure that personnel dealing with the inspection team are able to accurately and effectively answer questions that may be posed by FDA, and ensure that personnel are prepared to facilitate the conduct of the inspection by having key documents readily available. Emphasis was given to the importance of providing timely and appropriate response after inspections when FDA-483s have been issued. Practical ways to improve the chances of having a successful PAI were also included. FDA contacts were provided, as well as information useful for the successful completion of a foreign FDA PAI, hopefully leading to application approval.

Finally, a brief review of FDA enforcement practices was offered, because many companies continue to experience difficulties during PAIs. Four of the primary enforcement options were described, including nonapproval of applications, warning letters, Import Detentions, and the AIP. The authors believe that companies can significantly improve the odds of a successful PAI by using systematic techniques to prepare before the FDA arrives and by making certain personnel know what to expect. It appears that the FDA will continue an aggressive PAI program for the foreseeable future, including priority attention at international sites that manufacture APIs and finished drug products. Hopefully, the information presented here will be of value to those who expect to undergo a PAI at an international site.

APPENDIX 1: SELECTED FDA GUIDELINES, GUIDES AND GUIDANCE DOCUMENTS RELATED TO PAIs

Sources

The following are selected documents that have been published by the FDA in recent years on issues that are likely to be covered during PAIs, and are available from the following sources:

1. Freedom of Information (FOI) staff
   Food and Drug Administration,
   FOI Staff (HFI-35)
   5600 Fishers Lane, Rockville, Md. 20857
   Telephone: (301) 443-6310
   Facsimile: (301) 443-1726
2. CDER
   Food and Drug Administration,
   Center for Drug Evaluation and Research (CDER)
   (HFD-19),
   5600 Fishers Lane, Rockville, Md. 20857

Telephone: (301) 443-8491
Facsimile: (301) 594-5491
Fax on Demand: (301) 827-0577; 1 (800) 342-2722
Website: http:/www/fda.gov/cder

3. CBER
   Food and Drug Administration,
   Center for Biological Evaluation and Research (CBER)
   FOI Branch (HFM-48)
   5600 Fishers Lane, Rockville, Md. 20857
   Telephone: (301) 827-3817
   Facsimile: (301) 443-1726
   Fax on Demand: (301) 827-3844; 1 (888) 223-7329
   Website: http:/www/fda.gov/cber

Laws

Federal Food Drug and Cosmetic Act, as amended.

Public Health Service (PHS) Act

Regulations

21 CFR 211 Part 211, April 1996

21 CFR Part 314.70, A Supplements and Other Changes to an Approved Application

21 CFR Part 314.80, Annual Report

21 CFR Part 314.81, Other Postmarketing Reports (NDA field alert report)

21 CFR Part 11, Electronic Signatures; Electronic Records, Final Rule, Federal Register, Vol. 62, pp. 13431–13466, March 20, 1997

21 CFR Part 211, Current Good Manufacturing Practice, Amendment of Certain Requirements for Finished Pharmaceuticals, Proposed Final Rule, Federal Register, Vol. 61, pp. 20104–20115, May 3, 1996

Federal Register, Vol. 43, No. 190, pp. 45014–45089, Human and Veterinary Drugs, Current Good Manufacturing Practice in Manufacture, Processing, Packing, or Holding, September 29, 1978

Guidelines, Guides to Inspection, and Guidance Documents

1997

"Design Control Guidance for Medical Device Manufacturers" (March 11, 1997)

"Guidance for Industry—Manufacturing Equipment Addendum to the Guidance for Industry for Scale-Up and Post-Approval Changes: Immediate-Release Products," (SUPAC-IR) (February 1997)

1996

"Guidance for Industry: Manufacture, Processing or Holding of Active Pharmaceutical Ingredients," (August 1996)

"DRAFT Guidance for Industry, Modified Release Solid Oral Dosage Forms; Scale-Up and Post Approval Changes: Chemistry, Manufacturing and Controls, *In Vitro* Dissolution Testing, and *In Vivo* Bioequivalence Documentation," (June 7, 1996)

"Guide to Inspection of Infectious Disease Marker Testing Facilities," (June 1996)

"Guide to Inspections of Foreign Pharmaceutical Manufacturers," (May 1996)

"Guide to Inspections of Foreign Medical Device Manufacturers," (May 1996)

"BPC Process Validation" (March 1996)

"Content and Format for Submission of Drug Products for Investigational New Drug Applications (INDs), New Drug Applications (NDAs), Abbreviated New Drug Applications (ANDAs), and Abbreviated Antibiotic New Drug Applications," (February 1996)

"Changes to an Approved Application for Well-Characterized Therapeutic Recombinant DNA-Derived and Monoclonal Antibody Biotechnology Products," (January 1996)

1995

"Immediate Release Solid Oral Dosage Forms; Scale-Up and Postapproval Changes: Chemistry, Manufacturing, and Controls; *In Vitro* Dissolution Testing; *In Vivo* Bioequivalence Documentation; Guidance; Notice," (November 30, 1995)

"Guidance for Industry for the Submission of an Environmental Assessment in Human Drug Applications and Supplements," (November 1995)

"Guidance For Industry—Content and Format of Investigational New Drug Applications (INDs) for Phase I Studies of Drugs, Including Well-Characterized, Therapeutic, Biotechnology-Derived Products," (November 1995)

"Glossary of Computerized System and Software Development Terminology," (August 1995)

"International Conference on Harmonisation; Draft Guideline on Good Clinical Practice; Availability," (August 1995)

"Guidance for Development of Vaginal Contraceptive Drugs," (April 1995)

"Drug Registration And Listing Instruction Booklet," (February 1, 1995)

1994

"Supplements to New Drug Applications, Abbreviated New Drug Applications, or Abbreviated Antibiotic Applications for Nonsterile Drug Products; Draft Guideline," Federal Register, Vol. 59, pp. 64094–64096, (December 12, 1994)

"Guide to Inspections of Source Plasma Establishments," (December 1994)

"Draft Guideline on Supplements to NDAs, ANDAs, or AADAs for Nonsterile Drug Products," (December 1994)

"Interim Guidance, Immediate Release Solid Oral Doage Forms; Pre- And Post-Approval Changes: Chemistry, Manufacturing and Controls, *In Vitro* Dissolution Testing, and *In Vivo* Bioequivalence Documentation," (November 29, 1994)

"Interim Inactive Ingredients Policy," (November 1994)

"Reviewer Guidance—Validation of Chromatographic Methods," (November 1994)

"CANDA—Computer Assisted New Drug Application Guidance Manual," (October 1994)

"ORA Warning Letter Guide," (October 1994)

"Guidance for Industry—Format and Content for the CMC Section of an Annual Report," (September 1994)

"Guideline for Industry Stability Testing of New Drug Substances and Products," (September 1994)

"Guide to Inspections of Blood Banks," (September 1994)

"International Conference on Harmonisation; Stability Testing of New Drug Substances and Products; Guideline; Availability; Notice," (September 1994)

"Guide to Sterile Inspections of Oral Solutions and Suspensions," (August 1994)

"Guide to Inspections of Topical Drug Products," (July 1994)

"Guide to Inspections of Sterile Drug Substance Manufactures," (July 1994)

"Draft Points-to-Consider for OTC Actual-Use Studies," (July 1994)

"FDA/ORA Foreign Inspetion Manual and Travel Guide," FDA, Division of Field Investigations, ORA, (June 1994)

"Guide To Inspections of Bulk Pharmaceutical Chemicals," (May 1994)

"Guidance to Expedite the Review of Launch Campaign Submissions," (March 1994)

"A Guide to Inspections of Oral Solid Dosage Forms Pre/Post Approval Issues for Development and Validation," (January 1994)

1993

"Recommendations for Submitting Documentation for Sterilization Process Validation," FDA, Federal Register, Vol. 58, pp. 63996–64001 (December 12, 1993)

"Guideline for Adverse Experience Reporting For Licensed Biological Products," (October 1993)

"A Guide to Inspections of Dosage Form Drug Manufacturers—CGMPs," (October 1993)

"A Guide to Inspections of Validation of Cleaning Processes," (July 1993)

"A Guide to Inspections of Pharmaceutical Quality Control Laboratories," (July 1993)

"A Guide to Inspections of Microbiological Pharmaceutical Quality Control Laboratories," (July 1993)

"A Guide to Inspections of High Purity Water Systems," (July 1993)

"A Guide to Inspections of Lyophilization of Parenterals," (July 1993)

"New Drug Evaluation Guidance Document: Refusal to File," (July 1993)

"Guidance for Quality Assurance in Blood Establishments," (June 1993)

"FDA Guide for Detecting Fraud in Bioresearch Monitoring Inspections," (April 1993)

"A Guideline on Laboratory Acceptance Testing (Draft)," (March 1993)

"Guide to Inspection of Solid Oral Dosage Form Drug Manufacturing," (March 1993)

"Guide to Inspection of Solid Oral Dosage Form Validation Activities," (March 1993)

1992

"Conduct of Clinical Investigations: Responsibilities of Clinical Investigators and Monitors for Investigational New Animal Drug Studies," (October 1992)

"A Guide to Inspections of Foreign Pharmaceutical Manufacturing Plants," (September 14, 1992)

"Points to Consider in the Preclinical Development of Immunomodulatory Drugs for the Treatment of HIV Infection and Associated Disorders," (September 1992)

"Inspection Guide Pharmaceutical Quality Control, Laboratory," (June 22, 1992)

"Guideline for Postmarketing Reporting of Adverse Drug Experiences," (March 1992)

"Draft Guideline on Repackaging of Solid Oral Doage Form Drug Products," (1992)

"Mid-Atlantic Regional Inspection Guide for the Lyophilization of Parenterals," (1992)

1991

"Biotechnology Inspection Guide," (November 1991)

"Draft Guideline for Submitting Supporting Chemistry Documentation in Radiopharmaceutical Drug Applications," (November 1991)

"Guideline for Manufacture of In-Vitro Diagnostic Products," (October 1991)

"Guide to Inspections of Bulk Pharmaceutical Chemicals," (September 1991)

"Fraud, Untrue Statements of Material Facts, Bribery, and Illegal Gratuities; Final Policy," Federal Register, Vol. 56, No. 175, Docket 90N–0332, (September 10, 1991)

"Points to Consider in the Preparation of IND Applications for New Drugs Intended for the Treatment of HIV-Infected Individuals," (September 1, 1991)

"Reviewer Guidance for Computer Controlled Medical Devices Undergoing 510(k) Review," (August 1991)

"Points to Consider for Internal Reviews and Corrective Action Operating Plans," (June 1991)

"Guideline on the Preparation of Investigational New Drug Products (Human and Animal)," (March 1991)

1990

"FDA Center for Veterinary Medicine Drug Stability Guidelines," (December 1990)

"Application of the Medical Device GMPs to Computerized Devices and Manufacturing Processes—Medical Device GMP Guidance for FDA Investigators," (November 1990)

"Points to Consider in the Preclinical Development of Antiviral Drugs," (November 1990)

"Draft Guideline for Abuse Liability Assessment," (July 1990)

"Reviews of ANDAs/AADAs and DMFs," (May 1990)

"Guidelines for the Manufacture of In-Vitro Diagnostic Products," (February 1990)

"Mid Atlantic Region Pharmaceutical Inspection Program, Inspection Guidance for Prescription Drug Plants," (January 1990)

1989

"Guideline for Drug Master Files," (September 1989)

"Compressed Medical Gases Guideline," (February 1989)

1988

"Draft—Biotech Inspection Outline," (August 1988)

"Guideline for the Format and Content of the Clinical and Statistical Sections of New Drug Applications," (July 1988)

1987

"Guideline on Validation of the Limulus Amebocyte Lysate Test as an End-Product Endotoxin Test for Human and Animal Parenteral Drugs, Biological Products, and Medical Devices," (December 1987)

"Guide to Inspection of Bulk Pharmaceutical Chemical Manufacturing," (November 1987)

"Technical Report: Software Development Activities, Reference Materials and Training Aids for Investigators," (July 1987)

"Guideline on General Principles of Process Validation," (May 1987)

"Guideline on Sterile Drug Products Produced by Aseptic Processing," (June 1987)

"Guideline for Submitting Documentation for the Stability of Human Drugs and Biologics," (February 1987)

"Guideline for the Format and the Content of the Human Pharmacokinetics and Bioavailability Section of an Application," (February 1987)

"Guideline for Submitting Supporting Documentation in Drug Applications for the Manufacture of Drug Substances," (February 1987)

"Guideline for Submitting Supporting Documentation for the Manufacture of and Controls for Drug Products," (February 1987)

"Guideline for the Format and Content of the Microbiology Section of an Application," (February 1987)

"Guideline for the Format and Content of the Chemistry, Manufacturing and Controls Section of an Application," (February 1987)

"Guideline for the Format and Content of the Summary for New Drug and Antibiotic Applications," (February 1987)

"Guideline on Formatting, Assembling, and Submitting New Drug and Antibiotic Applications," (February 1987)

"DRLs Drug Establishment Registration and Drug Listing Instruction Booklet," (February 1987)

"Guideline for Submitting Samples and Analytical Data for Methods Validations," (February 1987)

"Guideline for Submitting Documentation for Packaging for Human Drugs and Biologics," (February 1987)

"Guideline for Submitting Samples and Analytical Data for Methods Validation," (February 1987)

"Guideline for the Format and Content of the Nonclinical/Pharmacology/Toxicology Section of an Application," (February 1987)

"Submission in Microfiche of the Archival Copy of an Application," (February 1987)

"Guideline on Formatting, Assembling, and Submitting New Drug and Antibiotic Applications," (February 1987)

"Guideline for Submitting Documentation for Packaging for Human Drugs and Biologics," (February 1987)

"Guideline for the Format and Content of the Summary for New Drug and Antibiotic Applications," (February 1987)

1984 and Before

"Validation of Solid Oral and Topical Dosage Forms," (1985)

"Draft Guideline for Stability Studies for Human Drugs and Biologics," (March 1984)

"Division Guidelines for the Evaluation of Controlled Release Drug Products," (March 18, 1984)

"Guide to Inspection of Bulk Pharmaceutical Chemical Manufacturing," (April 1984)

"Draft Guideline for Submission of Supportive Analytical Data for Methods Validation in New Drug Applications," (April 1984)

"Draft Guideline for Packaging for Human Drugs and Biologics," (January 1984)

"Guide to Inspection of Computerized Systems in Drug Processing," (February 1983)

"Draft Guideline for Validation of the Limulus Amebocyte Lysate Test as an End-Product Endotoxin Test for Human and Animal Parenteral Drugs, Biological Products, and Medical Devices," (February 1983)

"Inspectional Guideline for Bulk Pharmaceutical Chemicals," (April 1980)

"General Guidelines for OTC Drug Combination Products," (September 1978)

Compliance Policy Guide (CPG) Manual

The FDA's CPG manual contains a collection of policies on various topics. The following are selected examples (number and title) that pertain to pharmaceuticals and FDA inspection issues that might be covered during PAI inspections.

Chapter 32: Drugs—General Policies

7132.01: Class I Recalls of Prescription Drugs (10/01/80)

7132.02: Compendium Revisions and Deletions (10/01/80)

7132.03: Drugs—Declaration of Quantity of Active Ingredient by Both Metric and Apothecary Systems (10/01/80)

7132.04(*): Candy "Pills"—Representation as Drug (*)See CPG 7105.10 (10/01/80)

7132.05: Performance of Tests for Compendial Requirements on Compendial Products (10/01/80)

7132.06: Hospital Pharmacies—Status as Drug Manufacturer (10/01/80)

7132.07: Drugs, Human—Failure to Register (10/01/80)

7132.08: Collection and Charitable Distribution of Drugs (10/01/80)

7132.09: Return of Unused Prescription Drugs to Pharmacy Stock (10/01/80)

7132.10: CGMP Enforcement Policy—OTC vs Rx Drugs (4/01/82)

7132.11: Prescription Drugs for Ships' Medicine Chests (10/01/80)

7132.12: Consistent Application of CGMP Determinations (4/01/81)

7132.13: Repacking of Drug Products—Testing/Examination Under CGMPs (07/01/81)

7132.14: Control and Accountability of Labeling Associated with Tamper-Resistant Packaging of Over-the-Counter Drug Products (03/01/83)

7132.15: Conditions Under Which Homeopathic Drugs May Be Marketed (05/31/88)

7132.16: Manufacture, Distribution, and Promotion of Adulterated, Misbranded, or Unapproved New Drugs for Human Use by State-Licensed Pharmacies (03/16/92)

Chapter 32a: Drugs—Adulteration Policies

7132a.01:   Interference with Compendial Tests (10/01/80)

7132a.02:   Controlled Release Dosage Form Drugs—Rate of Released of
              Active Ingredients (09/04/87)

7132a.03:   Adulteration of Drugs Under Section 501(b) and 501(c) of the
              Act. Direct Reference Seizure Authority for Adulterated Drugs
              Under Section 501(b) (05/01/92)

7132a.04:   Requirements for Expiration Dating and Stability Testing
              (09/04/87)

7132a.0:   Finished Dosage Form Drug Products in Bulk Containers—
              Application of Current Good Manufacturing Practice Regula-
              tions (09/04/87)

7132a.07:   Computerized Drug Processing; Input/Output Checking (09/04/87)

7132a.08:   Computerized Drug Processing; Identification of "Persons" on
              Batch Production and Control Records (09/04/87)

7132a.10:   Lack of Expiration Date or Stability Data (09/04/87)

7132a.11:   Computerized Drug Processing; CGMP Applicability to Hard-
              ware and Software (09/04/87)

7132a.12:   Computerized Drug Processing; Vendor Responsibility (09/04/87)

7132a.13:   Parametric Release of Terminally Heat Sterilized Drug Products
              (10/21/87)

7132a.14:   Content Uniformity Testing of Tables and Capsules (10/02/87)

7132a.15:   Computerized Drug Processing; Source Code for Process Con-
              trol Application Programs (04/16/87)

7132a.15:   Compressed Medical Gases—Warning Letters for Specific Vio-
              lations Covering Liquid and Gaseous Oxygen* (08/31/92)

7132a.17:   Tamper-Resistant Packaging Requirements for Certain Over-
              the-Counter (OTC) Human Drug Products (05/21/92)

Chapter 32b: Drugs—Misbranding Policies

7132b.01:   OTC Ear Drop Preparations (05/22/87)

7132b.02:   Fructose-Containing Drugs (05/22/87)

7132b.03:   Smoking Deterrents—Misbranding (05/22/87)

7125.09:	Over-the-Counter Sale of Injectable Animal Drugs (10/01/80)
7125.10:	Veterinarian Use of New Animal Drug Substances (10/01/80)
7125.11:	Drugs for Odor Control in Animals (12/19/89)
7125.12:	Anthelmintics (10/01/80)
7125.13:	Furazolidone and Nitrofurazone in Animal Feed (10/01/80)
7125.14:	Biological Drugs for Animal Use (10/01/80)
7125.15:	Chemical Sterilization of Animal Parenteral Drugs (10/01/80)
7125.16:	Oral Iron Products for Baby Pigs (12/01/82)
7125.17:	Animal Drugs for Euthanasia (10/01/80)
7125.18:	Ethylenediamine Dihydroiodide (EDDI) (03/01/86)
7125.19:	Reconditioning of New Animal Drugs Seized Under Section 501(a)(5) (10/01/80)
7125.20:	Availability of Bulk Chemicals for Animal Drug Use (10/01/80)
7125.21:	Animal Grooming Aids (10/01/80)
7125.22:	Streptomycin Residues in Cattle Tissues (10/01/80)
7125.23:	Dimethyl Sulfoxide (DMSO) for Animal Use (10/01/80)
7125.24:	Adequate Directions for Use (Species Designation)—Animal Drugs and Veterinary Devices (10/01/80)
7125.25:	Failure to Register Attachment A (10/01/80)
7125.26:	Lay Use of Veterinary Prescription Drugs (03/01/82)
7125.27:	Terminal Heat Sterilization of Veterinary Multi-Dose Parenterals Containing a Preservative (10/01/80)
7125.28:	Flea and Tick Collars Containing a Pesticide (10/01/80)
7125.29:	Illegal Sales of Veterinary Prescription Drugs—Direct Reference Authority for Regulatory Letter Issuance (02/10/89)
7125.30:	Teat Dips and Udder Washes for Dairy Cows and Goats (07/01/82)
7125.31:	Large Volume Parenterals (LVPs) for Animal Use (12/01/82)
7125.32:	Plastic Containers for Injectable Animal Drugs (01/01/83)

7125.33:   Chloramphenicol as an Unapproved New Animal Drug—Direct Reference Seizure Authority (04/25/89)

7125.34:   Orders for Post-Approval Records Review (06/25/92)

7125.35:   Human-Labeled Drugs Distributed and Used in Animal Medicine (07/20/92)

7125.36:   Unapproved New Animal Drugs—Followup Action to Approved Regulatory Letter-Direct Reference Seizure Authority (04/16/91)

7125.37:   Proper Drug Use and Residue Avoidance by Non-Vets (07/09/93)

7125.38:   Process Validation Requirements for Drug Products Subject to Pre-Market Approval (08/30/93)

7125.39:   Drug Packaged for Infusion or Injection for Food-Producing Animals (08/23/94)

Letters and Policy Statements

1994

FDA Letter to ANDA and AADA Applicants dated April 8, 1994, Office of Generic Drugs (Douglas L. Sporn) [ID FDA 09144]

1993

FDA Letter to ANDA and AADA Applicants dated August 4, 1993, Office of Generic Drugs (Douglas Sporn) [ID FDA 09713]

1991

FDA Letter to Registered Drug Establishments dated November 3, 1991, regarding generic drug NDA submissions (Roger Williams) [ID FDA 06928]

FDA Internal Memorandum dated October 18, 1991, "Subject: Change in Policy—Validation of Processes Prior to Validation" (Richard Davis) [ID FDA 06931]

Transcript of Proceedings, Questions and Answers, FDA/Industry forums held during October/December 1991 in Cherry Hill, San Francisco, Chicago, and San Juan, (August 1992) [ID FDA 06943]

1990

Dr. Carl Peck Letter to All NDA and ANDA Holders and Applicants, dated June 1, 1990 (Carl Peck [ID FDA 06930]

Division of Generic Drug Policy and Procedures Guides (PPGs)

Summary listing division of generic drugs policy and procedure guides (PPG no. and subject).

1995

42-95:   Random Assignment of Original Applications and Related Documents to Bioequivalence Reviewers (June 9, 1995)

41-95:   Guidance on the Packaging of Test Batches (February 8, 1995)

1994

40-94:   Scoring Configuration of Generic Drug Products (December 15, 994)

39-94:   Random Assignment of Original Applications to Chemistry Reviewers (March 8, 1994)

1993

38-93:   Restatement of the Office of Generic Drugs' "First-In, First-Reviewed" Policy and Modification of the Exceptions to the Policy Regarding Minor Amendments (January 13, 1993)

1992

37-92:   Management of Office and Center Committees (October 15, 1992)

36-92:   Submission of an "Investigational New Drug Application" to the Office of Generic Drugs (OGD) (October 13, 1992)

35-92:   Revision of Exhibit Batch Requirements for Abbreviated Antibiotic Drug Applications (AADAs) (July 13, 1992)

34-92:   Implementation of the Fraud, Untrue Statements of Material Facts, Bribery, and Illegal Gratuities Final Policy (October 3, 1992)

33-92:   Consistent Container Information in an Abbreviated Application (February 24, 1992)

32-92:   Reaffirmation of Expiration Dating Period for Abbreviated Applications (January 14, 1992)

1991

31-91: Drug Master File (DMF) Reviews: Policy and Procedures (Revision to January 11, 1994)

30-91: Organization of an Abbreviated New Drug Application and an Abbreviated Antibiotic Application (April 10, 1991)

1990

29-90: Previously Reviewed Material in ANDA's, AADA's and DMF's with Respect to Reassigned Cases (Sepetember 20, 1990)

28-90: Subject: Issuance of Not-Approvable Letters on Originals and Supplements to ANDA's and AADA's (September 19, 1990)

27-90: Acceptance for Filing and Review of AADA's Absent Approval of the Referenced Bulk Antibiotic (September 13, 1990)

26-90: Reference to Type 1 Drug Master Files in ANDAs and AADAs Applications

25-90: Removal of Work Related Materials from the Division at the End of Employment (July 17, 1990)

24-90: Improvement by the Applicant of Unreviewed Original ANDA and AADA Submissions (July 31, 1990)

23-90: Submission of Reprocessing Procedures by ANDA and AADA Applicants (August 9, 1990)

22-90: Interim Policy on Exceptions to the Batch-Size and Production Condition Requirements for Non-Antibiotic, Solid, Oral-Dosage Form Drug Products Supporting Proposed ANDA's (September 13, 1990)

21-90: The "First In-First Reviewed" Policy and Exceptions Thereto as It Applies to Supplemental Applications to ANDAs and AADAs (May 22, 1990)

20-90: Variations in Solid Oral Dosage Forms and Injectables that Can be Included Within a Single ANDA (May 25, 1990)

19-90: Subject: Availability of Labeling Guidance (April 12, 1990)

18-90: Requests for Expedited Review of Supplements to Approved ANDA's and AADA's (January 22, 1992)

17-90: Issuance of Action Letters Within the Office of Generic Drugs (April 12, 1990)

16-90: The "First In-First Reviewed" Policy and Exceptions Thereto as It Applies to Original ANDA's and AADA's and Amendments (March 7, 1990)

15-90: Monitoring and Reporting the Progress of ANDA and AADA Reviews (January 18, 1990)

1989

14-89: Signatory Concurrence and Agreement on Final Typed Reviews and Letters and Other Items in the Administrative File (November 8, 1989)

13-89: Testing Requirements Applicable to Finished Dosage Forms Manufactured Outside the United States (November 2, 1989)

12-89: Number of Manufacturing Sites Permitted in an ANDA or AADA (November 2, 1989)

11-89: Shredding of Carbons, Draft Reviews and Letters (September 25, 1989)

10-89: Meetings with Pharmaceutical Firm Employees or Their Representatives (September 21, 1989)

9-89: Delivery of Documents to the Office of Generic Drugs' Document Room; Providing Requested Documents to Messengers and Other Representatives of ANDA/AADA Applicants (October 1, 1991)

8-89: Changes in Labeling of ANDAs Subsequent to Revision of Innovator Labeling (August 21, 1989)

7-89: Subject: Approvable Actions for ANDA and AADA Supplements (August 17, 1989)

6-89: Not Approvable Actions for ANDAs and Supplements (August 17, 1989)

5-89: Processing of Supplements that the Applicant Proposes to Put Into Effect Prior to Approval Under 21 CFR 314.70(C.) (August 13, 1989)

4-89: Microbiology Reviews of Abbreviated Applications (July 13, 1989, revised November 4, 1993)

3-89: Handling Telephone Inquiries on Status of Processing from Applicants or Their Representatives (August 1, 1989)

2-89: Batch Size Requirements for Drug Products Containing Controlled Substances and Inquiries to the Drug Enforcement Administration (August 1, 1989)

1-89: Subject: Correspondence Practices (July 13, 1989)

Compliance Program (CP) Manuals

CP 7346.832, Chapter 46—New Drug Evaluation, "Pre-Approval Audit Inspections," August 1994, and previous edition dated October 1, 1990 [ID FDA 06698 and 06750]

CP 7346.843, Chapter 46—New Drug Evaluation, "Post-Approval Audit Inspections," September 1994, and previous edition dated 1992 [ID FDA 07504]

CP 7356.002, Chapter 56—Drug Quality Assurance, "Drug Process Inspections," December 1990 [ID FDA 06431]

Compliance Program 7356.002a, Chapter 56—Drug Quality Assurance, "Sterile Drug Process Inspections," December 1990 [ID FDA 06431]

4

Stability Data and Pre-Approval Inspections

Christopher T. Rhodes
University of Rhode Island, Kingston, Rhode Island

I. INTRODUCTION

This chapter is specifically focused on stability data and pre-approval inspections. This very broad subject is often of substantial, if not critical, importance in pre-approval inspections and is given very considerable attention by Food and Drug Administration (FDA) investigators. Given the wide variety of drugs and dosage forms that the pharmaceutical industry produces, the range of potential problems in stability data is vast. The author of this chapter is well aware that he has not addressed all conceivable stability matters that could be involved in a pre-approval inspection—that would not be possible. However, it is hoped that the material in this chapter will at least provide a flavor of some of the aspects of stability that require attention and suggest possible procedures that may assist in optimizing interactions with FDA personnel. There are some matters that are touched on in this chapter that have broader implications than just stability aspects of pre-approval inspections. Thus, some of the topics discussed in this chapter apply, at least in part, to market batch evaluation and troubleshooting. In addition, stability considerations cannot be considered in isolation from the other chapters of this book, such as those authored by Dr. Nash (Chapter 7) or Dr. Wray (Chapter 6), which obviously impact on stability testing.

II. WHY DO WE ACCUMULATE STABILITY DATA

There are at least three major reasons why we accumulate stability data: (1) because we are required to do so by regulatory agencies; (2) to protect the reputation of our company as a producer of quality products; and (3) to obtain data that may be of value in the formulation and processing of other products (extending our scientific data base).

All three reasons are valid, and it may well be that in the development of stability data for a new product all three reasons may, to a greater or lesser extent, define the scope of stability studies. This is perfectly reasonable. What is unacceptable is the attitude, which may be perceived in some companies, where reason number one is regarded as the *only* justification of stability work. There are occasions when any reputable company will decide to embark on stability studies over and above the minimum defined by FDA or International Conference on Harmonization (ICH) requirements.

III. THE PRESENT REGULATORY STATUS WITH RESPECT TO STABILITY TESTING

In the United States, there is presently an interregnum between the 1987 FDA Guidelines [1] and the new ICH Guidelines [2] that become official in 1998. This situation creates uncertainty for those of us working for the U.S. pharmaceutical industry on drug product stability for several reasons.

First, the new ICH Guidelines are in some areas, considerably less specific than the 1987 FDA Guidelines. This means that there is probably more leeway for genuine dispute about interpretation. Second, we do not yet know how well or how poorly FDA investigators in districts throughout the United States will be knowledgeable about the content of the ICH Guidelines. Since in recent years a number of FDA observers have detected an increasing level of independence and variability in the activities of FDA districts, there may well be legitimate concern on this point. Third, until a period of 2 or 3 years has elapsed, we probably will not know with any degree of certainty how the FDA in Rockville, MD, intends to apply ICH, let alone how individual FDA districts will react.

In this time of flux, it is particularly important that we carefully watch for all official statements that the agency may issue concerning what is likely to be an evolving process on the development of precedents concerning the application of the ICH Guidelines. For example, obtaining data of 483's (Notice of Adverse Finding) concerning stability topics may well be of special value in this time of transition.

It is certainly important that those in the pharmaceutical industry who have responsibilities in stability make sure that they are fully conversant with the new ICH policies. The second edition of *Drug Stability: Principles and Practices* by the internationally renowned scientist, Jens Carstensen, is strongly recommended as a source of information on drug product stability and expiration dating [3].

The *FDA Compliance Program Guidance Manual* [4] specifically states:

> Product Stability: Inspection of the establishment to determine compliance with CGMP requirements and the validity of data supporting product stability and to conduct an audit of the data furnished to CDER in an application is a Field responsibility. This requirement applies both to the relevant preapproval batches, as discussed above, and the proposed commercial batches.

This is indeed a broad mandate and can allow investigation of a wide area. It is recommended that those concerned with stability should obtain, read, mark, learn, and inwardly digest the whole of this document. In addition, the Proposed Rule (May 3, 1996) for the Amendment to Current Good Manufacturing Procedures (CGMP) Regulations [5] and subsequent documents on CGMP should be examined.

It should be noted that the FDA Compliance Program Guidance of 1990 specifically states that preapproval inspections would be performed for the following categories: (1) drugs with a narrow therapeutic range; (2) new chemical entities; (3) generic versions of the 200 most prescribed drugs; (4) all cases where the plant and/or dosage form has not received a satisfactory inspection within the last 2 years; (5) when the application was the initial one for the application in question; and (6) all cases where the Center for Drug Evaluation and Research (CDER) review had disclosed discrepancies warranting further investigation.

Table 1 lists the drugs that appear in the FDA category of narrow therapeutic index or range. This list was originally defined as the list drugs for which the therapeutic ratio (LD50/ED50) is two or less. Drugs that appeared on the list were designated as ineligible for a bioavailability test waiver.

IV. POTENTIAL ADVERSE EFFECTS OF INSTABILITY IN PHARMACEUTICAL PRODUCTS

There is a misconception in the minds of some that stability testing is restricted to studies of potency. This is often far from the truth and, for some pharmaceutical products, there are quality attributes other than potency that are critical in stability

Table 1 Narrow Therapeutic Range Drugs

Aminophylline Tabs, ER Tabs
Carbamazepine Tabs, Oral Suspension
Clindamycin HCl Caps
Clonidine HCl Tabs
Clonidine Transdermal
Dyphylline Tabs
Disopyramide Phosphate Caps, DR Caps
Ethinyl Estradiol/Progestin Oral Contraceptive Tabs
Quanethidine Sulfate Tabs
Isoetherine Mesylate Inhalation Aerosol
Isoproterenol HCl Inhalation Aerosol
Lithium Carbonate Camsp, Tabs, ER Tabs
Metaproterenol Sulfate Tabs
Minoxidil Tabs
Oxtriphylline Tabs, DR Tabs, ER Tabs
Phenytoin Sodium Caps (Prompt or Extended), Oral Suspension
Prazopin HCl Caps
Primidene Tabs, Oral Suspension
Procainamide HCl Caps, Tabs, ER Tabs
Quinidine Sulfate Caps, Tabs, ER Tabs
Quinidine Gluconate Tabs, ER Tabs
Theophylline Caps, ER Caps, Tabs, ER Tabs
Valproic Acid Caps, Syrup
Vivalproex Sodium, DR Caps, DR Tabs
Warfarin Sodium Tabs

DR, delayed release; ER, extended release.

testing. This "potency of view" can cause difficulties with the FDA either with the CDER or during a pre-approval inspection. Rather than restrict our focus just to potency, we should have a concern for any functionally relevant quality attribute of the product that may change with time.

Some adverse effects of drug product instability that may merit attention in a stability program include the following: (1) loss of active (potency); (2) increase in concentration of active; (3) alteration of bioavailability; (4) loss of content uniformity; (5) decline in microbiological status; (6) increase in possibly toxic decomposition product; (7) loss of pharmaceutical elegance; and (8) modification in any other factor of functional relevance (e.g., loss of adhesion strength in a transdermal).

V. STABILITY DATA THAT SHOULD BE AVAILABLE AT THE TIME OF A PRE-APPROVAL INSPECTION

A. Adequate Test Methods

The sponsor of a new drug application (NDA), abbreviated new drug application (ANDA), or PLA should have available full, written descriptions of all the test methods that will be used in the stability program.

The quantification of active (potency) should be stability, indicating such that the drug can be separated from other components of the drug delivery system. The assay should also be capable of quantifying major degradation products.

For many products, tests for appearance are listed on stability test procedures. It is somewhat surprising to see the variability with which different companies apply such tests. At one extreme are tests that appear to consist, in essence, of a quick, untutored glance at the article in question by anyone who happens to be available. At the other end of the spectrum are meticulously conducted, objective studies, some of which are rigorously interpreted, using, when appropriate, nonparametric, statistical methods. Not surprisingly, the appearance tests of the first type in some companies always gain a designation of "satisfactory," whereas those of the second are more likely to reveal possible problems. The devaluation of appearance tests is to be regretted since, for some products, careful evaluation of appearance can be of considerable value in a stability program. For example, if an emulsion that is initially white shows a tendency to turn slightly yellow on storage, this may well be an indication of physical or microbiological instability. Careful comparison of the product with standard color charts will reveal this subtle change; quick, noncomparative, purely subjective evaluations probably will not.

Obviously, in selecting test methods for a stability program, one should try to select those that are steadily reproducible and precise. Thus, in general, we should reduce our reliance on bioassays and convert to physicochemical-type assays (such as high-performance liquid chromatography [HPLC]) as much as possible. This consideration will, of course, be of particular importance when we are working with peptides or proteins; but even for micromolecular drugs, this issue can be important. For example, if it is intended to measure preservative efficacy as part of a stability protocol, it may be appropriate to use a chemical assay as the test method on all stations except the last test, when the United States Pharmacopeia (USP) Preservative Challenge test would be used.

B. Validation Data for Test Methods

The validation of stability-indicating, analytical methods designed for use in the stability protocol is highly likely to be subjected to considerable scrutiny during a pre-approval inspection. It is therefore essential that considerable care be directed to preparing this area for examination by FDA personnel. Because of the critical nature of assay validation documentation, "dry runs" or self-audit inspections by a company's own employees are especially valuable for assay validation.

To obtain maximum value from an in-house, self-audit inspection conducted in advance of actual FDA pre-approval inspection, it is imperative that the planning, operation, and review of the results be treated very seriously by all concerned. If deficiencies are revealed during the self-audit, top priority must be given to taking all appropriate remedial action. Depending on the nature of the problem, it may be necessary to: (1) perform additional laboratory studies; (2) conduct an investigation of the problem and issue a report that will be kept on file and made available to FDA personnel should they so request; and/or (3) modify standard operating procedures (SOPs) to require training, purchase of new equipment, etc.

The necessity not only of the initial validation of a stability-indicating assay, but also of a continuing process of assuring that the stability-indicating assay remains approximately validated throughout the period of its use must be kept in mind. There are occasions when the specific requirements with respect to assay validation as expounded by the FDA should be exceeded. For example, even if it is known that an official method is stability indicating, it is my belief that it is prudent to have some in-house validation data on how the method performs in our laboratory, despite the statement by the FDA [5]: "Compendial methods . . . reflect years of experience and evaluation and in most cases do not need to be revalidated." Among the key official documents pertinent to assay validation are the relevant general chapters of USP, ICH Guidelines on Validation of Analytical Procedures, and the FDA Reviewer Guidance—Validation of Chromatographic Methods [6,7]. These documents and other material available in the public domain give an excellent background on the principles and practices of assay validation with respect to physicochemical methods.

The FDA has stated [7]:

> Laboratory equipment and procedures must be quantified and validated. Every NDA/ANDA inspection will include an evaluation of laboratory controls and procedures and an audit of some of the raw data used to generate results. This data may be located in research and development test logs. The authenticity and accuracy of data used in the development of a test method should be reviewed. Use the Guide to Inspection of Pharmaceutical Quality Control Laboratories, July 1993, for inspectional criteria when covering laboratory operations.

These statements, and others in the document, make it clear that investigators have a broad mandate to inspect a wide range of data. In addition, although the Reviewer Guidance [7] states:

> CDER application review chemists are responsible for the review of the proposed drug product stability protocol, specifications and evaluation of the data submitted in support of the expiration dating period proposed for the drug product in the application

it would be imprudent for the sponsors of an NDA or ANDA not to be prepared for some pre-approval inspections to involve, tangentially at least, some of these broader issues.

For regulatory purposes, the 1987 Guideline defined stability-indicating methodology as:

> Quantitative analytical methods that are based on the characteristic structural, chemical or biological properties of each active of a drug product and that will distinguish each active ingredient from its degradation products so that the active ingredient content can be accurately measured.

However, as has already been noted, we have now extended our definition of stability-indicating assays to include the ability, where appropriate, to quantify some degradation products.

1. Characterization of Drug Substance

For those conducting a pre-approval inspection, one of the first foci of attention may well be the characterization of the drug substance and the specifications of the materials used in the preparation of standards and controls used in stability-indicating assays. For an ANDA submission, this question is normally readily disposed of; the sponsor will designate the use of a USP Reference Standard as the primary reference standard. The USP has developed a fine reputation for supplying a wide range of reproducible, quality reference products that are used not only in North America, but also in many other parts of the world. The only complaint that concerns these products is that they cannot be described as cheap in any sense of the word. However, to reduce costs, it is, of course, common practice to use an in-house standard, calibrated against the USP standard for much of the analytical work.

For the sponsor of an NDA that applies to a new chemical entity (NCE), it is highly improbable that a USP reference standard will be available. This will often mean that the sponsor must characterize the drug substance, impurities, and degradation pathways such that a reliable, in-house standard can be developed. Data supporting the reliability of this standard must be available. When the NCE is a macromolecule, the problems involved in this task can become very substantial. Even when, as is common, a battery of sophisticated test methods are used in attempts to fully characterize a protein, there will be occasions when, in reality, our ultimate reference is quantification of biological responses, which is notoriously imprecise.

2. Calibration of Equipment

Since the reliability of a stability-indicating assay often depends, to a significant extent, on the calibration of equipment used in the assay, it is by no means unreasonable for FDA investigators to give attention to this topic when conducting a pre-approval inspection. This matter should never be a problem. Unfortunately, however, it sometimes gets overlooked. Calibration of stability chambers is a hot topic for some FDA investigators (see Section VII.F).

3. Less Common Assay Validation Parameters

Most pharmaceutical scientists with responsibilities for assay validation are well aware of the type of data normally required for assay validation [8–11]. Parameters that may require attention include: accuracy, limit of detection, limit of quantification, linearity, precision, range, recovery, robustness, sample stability (on storage and during assay), specificity and selectivity, and systems suitability. Two additional parameters that may need special attention are transferability and comparability.

Transferability of an assay is the term applied to the differences or equivalence that may be detected when the same analytical procedure is performed at different locations (possibly in different countries). Thus, it is a form of robustness. Transferability studies may involve work by different analysts, using perhaps slightly different types of equipment, in facilities where environmental controls (e.g., temperature and relative humidity) may show substantial variance.

Comparability of an assay is required when it is decided to substitute a nonofficial assay method for an official test method, such as one specified by the USP. Comparability studies should clearly demonstrate that the assay parameters (accuracy, precision, etc.) of the test method to be used are at least as good, if not better, than those that characterize the official method.

4. Revalidation

There is a misconception in some quarters that once a stability-indicating method has been validated, there is no need for further validation. This is rarely, if ever, true. First, the method often evolves by small, incremental changes in solvents, guard columns, equipment, etc. Second, and in many cases more importantly, the level of expertise and dedication of the analysts often change significantly. The question that often arises is: "When should a method be revalidated?" The Canadian Health Protection Branch (HPB) has issued a document [12] that states:

> At least partial revalidation is required whenever significant changes are made either in the method itself or in the material analyzed, which could reasonably be expected to affect the results obtained (e.g., changes in equipment or suppliers of critical supplies).

Any change in the performance of an assay (e.g., changes in the slope or intercept of the calibration curve) should be a red flag, alerting those in charge of the assay of the possible need for partial revalidation. Even in the absence of such signals, it is probably prudent to consider some type of partial revalidation exercise at least once a year.

5. Physical Test Methods

Many of the examples referred to in the literature on assay validation relate specifically to HPLC or other chromatographic techniques. Of course, such methods are very common; unfortunately, however, the lack of reference to other techniques may seem to imply that assay validation only applies to physico-chemical analytical methods. This is, of course, not true. Any method used in a stability-testing protocol should be validated as far as possible.

Unfortunately, the relative paucity of publications on test methods that can be used in the evaluation of physical characteristics of drug delivery systems is a distinct disadvantage. Thus, it may well be that in some cases, both development and validation of the assay will have to be entirely in-house, although the literature does contain reports of some physical tests, such as redispersibility and sedimentation volumes of suspensions [13].

6. Forced Degradation

For an NCE that requires the development of an entirely new stability-indicating assay, it will be necessary to demonstrate that procedure is indeed stability-indicating by forced degradation studies. The Guideline [8] requires:

> A degradation schematic for the active ingredient in the dosage form, where possible (e.g., products of acid/base hydrolysis, temperature degradation, photolysis, and oxidation).

Tables 2 and 3 provide some useful information on stress testing (note that these data were prepared before the advent of the new ICH Guidelines on photostability testing, which require light sources calibrated in lumens).

Table 2 Suggested Outline for Performing Forced Degradations: Decide/Select Matrix for Degradation

Product/matrix	Degradation conditions							
	Degradation	Acid	Base	Peroxide	Bisulfite	UV	Visible	Heat
Product	Yes	X	X	X	X	X	X	X
Placebo/vehicle	Yes	X	X	X	X	X	X	X
Drug substance/								
raw material	Yes	X	X	X	X	X	X	X
Internal standard	No	—	—	—	—	—	—	—
Blank solution	Yes	X	X	X	X	X	X	X
Controls								
Product	No	—	—	—	—	—	—	—
Drug/substance/								
raw material	No	—	—	—	—	—	—	—
Blank solution	No	—	—	—	—	—	—	—

Source: Hong, 1996.
UV, ultraviolet.

The idea of stress testing as an aid to demonstrating that an analytical procedure is indeed stability-indicating is useful, but it is not perfect. For example, there are some drugs, such as auric chloride, that are inherently stable, and thus studies of the effect of stress on these products will only be of limited value. In addition, for protein drugs, our often incomplete knowledge of the molecule is a barrier to completely reliable demonstration of the stability-indicating nature of the assay (or assays) that we intend to use in stability tests.

Table 3 Suggested Outline for Performing Forced Degradations: Decide/Select Degradation Conditions/Agents

Medium	Conditions
1 N HCl, 10 mL	Reflux 30 min
0.1 N NaOH, 10 mL	Reflux 30 min
3% Hydrogen peroxide, 10 mL	Reflux 30 min
10% Sodium bisulfite, 10 mL	Reflux 30 min
Light	1. UV (254 nm), UV box 7 days
	2. Visible (RT), 1000 ft candles, 7 days
Dry heat	80°C, 7 days

Source: Hong, 1996.
UV, ultraviolet; RT, room temperature.

C. Preformulation Studies, Bulk Drug Substance

As previously noted, the FDA has stated [7] that in a pre-approval inspection, "data may be located in research and development test logs." One section of such documents that pertains to stability is preformulation studies directed to the stability of the bulk drug substance alone or in model test systems. Unfortunately, it is true that even today the quality of record keeping by persons in pharmacy research and development is often distinctly lower than that observed by quality control/quality assurance (QC/QA) personnel. Thus, it may be especially useful in any self-audit exercise to direct particular attention to this area.

D. Standard Operating Procedures

During a pre-approval inspection, it is highly likely that FDA investigators will examine the SOPs that relate to the development and operation of the stability program. There are two main reasons for such examinations: (1) evaluation of SOPs can often give a good idea of the strengths and weaknesses of a stability program; and (2) investigators will often be interested in seeing to what extent, if any, there are discrepancies between what a company says it will do in stability studies and how it actually performs. Unfortunately, there are often instances in which there are significant differences, and there are occasions when a company may be totally unable to give any rational explanation of the cause of the discrepancy. When outside consultants or FDA investigators find that the only place where SOPs are available is in the QC/QA manager's office, an alarm bell is likely to be activated in their minds. Although it is indeed appropriate that the QC/QA manager and other executives have copies of SOPs, it is essential that SOPs be readily available in the laboratory where the specified task is to be performed. If SOPs are not available at these locations, the possibility of the discrepancies previously referred to will be significantly increased.

It is, of course, important that SOPs be updated on a regular basis and that those who actually perform the task that is described in any given SOP be provided with an adequate opportunity to give input concerning possible modifications.

Although the general quality of SOPs used in the pharmaceutical industry has improved significantly in the last decade, there are still examples of verbosity and ambiguity that provide the potential for confusion and regulatory problems.

E. Room Temperature and Accelerated Test Data

For products that will be labeled to require storage at controlled room temperature, long-term studies at 25°C ± 2°C with 60% relative humidity (RH; ± 5%) with at least 12 months data are needed. Accelerated studies at 40°C ± 2°C and 75% ± 5% RH with at least 6 months data are also normally required. However, the ICH does allow for a less rigorous accelerated test if the 40°C test cannot be passed. When "significant change" occurs during the 40°C accelerated study, an intermediate test, such as 30°C ± 2°C and 60% RH ± 5% for 12 months, can be used. Significant change is defined as a 5% loss of potency, exceeding pH limits, dissolution failure, and failures of physical specifications (hardness, color, etc.).

If products are to be labeled with instructions for storage at a temperature of less than 25°C, then the accelerated studies can be performed at a temperature less than 40°C; however, the conditions should be at least 15°C above those used for long-term evaluation.

Products for which water loss may be more important, such as liquids or semisolids in plastic containers, it can be appropriate to replace high RH conditions by lower RH, such as 10% to 20%.

If, during clinical trials, a number of different formulations have been used that differ in either formulation or processing variables from the product intended for the market, it may be appropriate to "build bridges" between the various formulations if there is reason to believe that the changes in the formulation or processing variables are such that might reasonably be expected to significantly modify stability. The FDA SUPAC (scale-up and post-approval changes) Guideline may be of value in reaching a decision about the importance of such changes.

F. Data Concerning Contract Laboratory Stability Testing

The practice of using the services of an outside contract testing laboratory for part or all of the stability testing has become more common in recent years. Obviously, the quality of the data generated at such a facility is a matter of legitimate concern. It is also important to have documentation available that demonstrates the process that was used to select the particular testing laboratory; the evaluation of the contract laboratory's facilities, equipment, personnel, procedures, etc.; the instructions given to the contractor; and the mechanism of supervision, audit, and communication with the contractor.

VI. SPECIAL TREATMENT OF STABILITY DATA

A. Proteins

The stability testing of macromolecular drugs is often a most challenging risk. For some such drugs, our knowledge of the active drug may not be complete, although a number of different physicochemical and biological tests may have been used in our attempts to characterize the molecule. In addition, the fact that the degradation pathways for macromolecules can be complex and not easy to define fully can be an additional complication. It is also common during the development stage of a macromolecular drug for the primary assay method used to quantify potency to be a bioassay. Such methods are usually characterized by low precision, even when an extensive number of replicates are used; thus, attempts to use such methods to predict shelf life may be fraught with uncertainty. Indeed, any estimate of the time taken for a 10% loss of activity may well have a very substantial error associated with it. There is no easy or universal solution to this problem. One method that can be of value in assigning an expiration data for molecular drugs is to develop, as soon as possible, an in vitro bio-response assay that will usually have much better precision than a regular bioassay. For example, for epidermal growth factor, measurement of percentage of epidermal cells in mitosis is likely to be much more precise than the somewhat notorious hog wounding assay. The clot lysis assay for TPA is another example of an in vitro bio-response assay that has reasonable precision. Although such assays may not, at the commencement of marketing, be the primary assay for potency, there can be value in using them for shelf-life determinations.

Because the stability of a protein drug can often present new and unexpected challenges, it may well be an appropriate early stage of the drug's development to have a meeting in Rockville, MD, with appropriate FDA personnel to explain the strategy that the sponsor intends to use in the stability testing program. A record of the meeting, including any suggestions or comments made by FDA personnel, should be readily available at the time of the pre-approval inspection.

B. ANDAs

In general, developing stability data for an ANDA product will involve fewer laboratory studies than those required when an NCE is the subject of our studies. However, there are some aspects of stability testing for ANDAs that do pose special problems. First, there have been comments made by a number of pharmaceutical scientists and regulators that the ICH Stability Guideline appears to have been specifically designed for NCEs, rather than for ANDAs and generic drugs. This alleged bias has, in the opinion of some, resulted in insufficient attention being given to ANDA-type products, with the result that there is some uncertainty as to exactly how ICH principles will, or should, be applied for generic products. Hopefully, in the very near future there will be additional clarification from the FDA that will assist ANDA sponsors.

Often, the stability objective for an ANDA-type product is to develop a product that has essentially the same stability attributes as those possessed by that of the innovating company. Thus, in the absence of any patent considerations that might direct the generic away from the methods used by the innovator, it will be common to use the innovator's product as the template for the stability of the ANDA product. (Of course, there is nothing to prevent an ANDA sponsor from trying to formulate a product with a longer shelf life than that of the innovator, and this idea has been considered by some companies.)

If there is a USP specification for the bulk phar..iaceutical drug substance, the generic company will require its supplier to provide a Certificate of Analysis stating that the material is of pharmacopoeial quality. It is prudent for the pharmaceutical company to conduct at least some tests on some batches to assure that the bulk drug substance is acceptable. Information on the source and quality of the drug substance may well be subject to evaluation during a pre-approval inspection. If the generic company is reliably informed that its supplier of the drug substance is the same as that used by the innovator, this will be a considerable advantage. However, it is not uncommon for the innovator to have a source of drug substance that is not available to the generic company. In this instance, it may be useful for the company to conduct a detailed comparison of the raw material that it plans to use with the USP reference standard, which is, of course, normally provided by the innovator. Any evidence of a different synthetic route or differences in degradation and/or impurities might stimulate the need for further study.

Time is a problem in the accumulation of stability data for all pharmaceutical products. This is especially true for ANDA products, since the time-consuming, preclinical, clinical, and other studies that are essential for an NDA are not required. Thus, for an ANDA, unlike an NDA, the time required for the stability testing may be the rate-deciding factor for the entire development process. Because FDA investigators are aware of this situation, the evaluation of the stability program for an ANDA may well become especially significant. Obviously, stability studies should start as soon as possible (at 25°C, 30°C, and 40°C), as soon as one or more potential, marketable formulations/processes are available. It is much better to "waste" resources testing the stability of products that ultimately will not reach commercialization, rather than waste time not starting stability studies until we are absolutely certain of the precise details of both the formulation and process for the market product. Even if this approach is used, there will be occasions when the formulation that is ultimately selected for market will show differences greater than that permitted by SUPAC, and thus comparative, accelerated testing will be needed to build bridges that demonstrate stability equivalence between products that entered at 25°C, 30°C, and 40°C at the start of the stability program, and those that entered at a later date. In such circumstances, it can be helpful for the sponsor to prepare a document that succinctly explains the rationale of a stability testing program and to have such material available for the pre-approval inspection.

Another problem for the sponsors of ANDAs is the relative paucity of valuable data in the literature for the validation of dissolution testing and other methodologies; however, there are signs that this situation is now changing [14].

Perhaps the two biggest problems that affect the stability program for ANDA products in some generic companies are: (1) the lack of statistical expertise; and (2) the pressure of work on the chemists responsible for the stability testing. The lack of statistical expertise can be addressed by encouraging one or more persons in QC/QA to obtain training in the relatively basic statistical techniques used in the stability testing of ANDA products. The book by Dr. Sandford Bolton is a most useful reference [15], that can be of assistance in this area. Persons with some competence in the application of statistics to stability testing should be made available to answer any questions on this topic that may arise during the pre-approval inspection.

The pressure on the chemists who have responsibility for generating stability test data may be addressed in several ways as may be appropriate for the circumstances of the individual company. In some cases, top management needs to be persuaded that the capacity of the laboratory is unacceptably small. Capacity can be improved either by increasing the level of automation or by hiring additional, suitably qualified employees. When stability test data are consistently obtained later than planned, this is a clear sign of either poor management or insufficient laboratory capacity. These matters should be firmly resolved in advance of any pre-approval inspection.

C. Problem Drugs

It is fortunate for those involved in stability studies that many of the drug substances and delivery systems with which we are involved are relatively standard in nature. They seldom present any unusual or unexpected challenge, and the FDA and ICH Guidelines normally provide a reasonable basis for dealing with such projects. However, from time to time, pharmaceutical scientists do work on "stability problem drugs." This category includes drugs that exhibit a variety of problems, including unusual degradation pathways, analytical difficulties, substantial interbatch variability, esoteric kinetics, or shortage of bulk drug substance. When working on unusual stability challenges of this type, it may well be appropriate to meet with FDA officials in Rockville, MD, to discuss the project and explain to the agency the approach that the sponsor intends to use in developing stability data for the NDA or other market approval documents.

When visiting the FDA to discuss some special stability problem, the following points should be kept in mind. It is neither appropriate nor advantageous for a sponsor simply to ask FDA personnel how to solve any given stability problem or design any stability protocol. This is not the FDA's responsibility. However, it is perfectly reasonable, and indeed prudent, to describe the special nature of the stability challenge being considered and the plan that the sponsor has developed to meet the challenge. Agency chemists may well suggest possible modifications to the proposed plan. After the meeting at the FDA, a letter should be sent from the sponsor to the FDA thanking the agency for the meeting and stating the sponsor's understanding of the consensus that was reached at the meeting. This letter, together with other relevant documents, should be readily available at the time of the pre-approval inspection. The importance of stability concerns for problem drugs and other categories is referred to by Cartright and Matthews [16] and Avalone [17].

D. Numbers of Samples

For some drugs at the development stage, there may be a shortage of drug substances, which can have an adverse impact on the number of stability samples that can be entered into the stability testing program. Faced by this problem, some pharmaceutical scientists have shown considerable ingenuity. For example, some have developed miniaturized container systems for their stability studies and have validated, by a comparative study, that conditions imposed by the use of such systems are equally, if not more, stressful than those imposed by the full-size containers. Another strategy that may be of value is to use nondestructive sample testing; near infrared spectroscopy has considerable potential in this area [18]. Perhaps the most useful approach at present for many pharmaceutical scientists faced with this problem is to use a fractional factorial design (bracketing); this topic is discussed in Section VII. Whatever strategy is used, it should be fully documented with adequate supporting data so that at the time of pre-approval inspection, the FDA investigators can be shown a clear paper trail.

E. Bracketing

Bracketing, or matrixing, is a form of partial factorial experimental design that is well established as a respectable approach to reducing the amount of experimental work required for investigating a multivariable system, often with surprisingly little reduction in the statistical power associated with the conclusion. For instance, Nakagaki presents an example of a drug product produced at three dosage levels (50, 75, and 100 mg) in four-pack (blister, 15, 100, and 500 pack) and three-pack materials [19]. If all possible combinations were examined in a stability program, we would perform 36 separate studies. However, it was suggested that only 18 such systems need to be tested, with samples of the remainder being available for testing should the need arise (Table 4). Many more elaborate experimental designs, some involving the reduction of tests at various testing

Table 4 Bracketing Stability Design

	Dosage strength/raw material lot								
	50 mg			75 mg			100 mg		
Packaging	A	B	C	A	B	C	A	B	C
Blister	X	X	X	(X)	(X)	(X)	X	X	X
HDPE/15 pack size	X	X	X	(X)	(X)	(X)	X	X	X
HDPE/100 pack size	(X)	(X)	(X)	(X)	(X)	(X)	(X)	(X)	(X)
HDPE/500 pack size	X	X	X	(X)	(X)	(X)	X	X	X

X, testing carried out; (X), testing not routinely carried out, although samples may still be retained for testing if needed; HDPE, high-density polyethylene bottle.

intervals, have been proposed. Care must be taken not to apply this approach in an invalid way. Thus, suppose that in the above example the formulation used for the 100-mg tablets was different from that used for the 50- and 75-mg tablets. It would not be appropriate to include all three formulations in one bracketed experimental design.

Since, as far as has been indicated to this author, the comfort level with respect to bracketing varies significantly within the FDA, it would probably be unwise for sponsors to embark on elaborate bracketing studies without having first checked with an appropriate FDA official concerning the acceptability of the proposed approach. Documentation concerning such discussions should be available at any pre-approval inspection, although it is likely that in time more regulatory agencies will regard bracketing as relatively standard [20].

VII. PROBLEMS TO AVOID IN RESPONDING TO QUESTIONS ON STABILITY DATA AT PRE-APPROVAL INSPECTIONS

A. Data Not Readily Retrievable

It is not unreasonable for an FDA investigator conducting a pre-approval inspection to expect to be able to examine any stability data pertinent to the inspection within a short time of making a request to the sponsor's employees. Unfortunately, the availability of such documents is not always optimal. Excluding such catastrophes as fire or tornadoes, it is usually hard to justify the difficulties in retrieving stability data. In these days of computerized record-keeping, such data should be easily obtainable in a very short period of time. As previously mentioned, a self-audit conducted before the FDA pre-approval inspection can be of value in identifying and remedying problems of this type.

B. Obscure, Aberrant, Incomplete, Failing, or Possibly Fraudulent Data

Usually, there is no valid excuse for a sponsor being "surprised" when an FDA investigator draws attention to what appears to be obscure, aberrant, incomplete, failing, or possibly fraudulent data during an FDA pre-approval inspection. The company should have identified any such potential during its self-audit process and taken appropriate remedial action. At the very least, such action should include the issuance of a report that recognizes the problem, explains (if possible) the cause, defines what corrective measures have been implemented, and presents a rational argument as to why it can be concluded that the effect of the possible problem is unsubstantial. When appropriate, a formal failure investigation should be completed [21].

C. Lack of One Person as Stability Coordinator with the Big Picture

The practice of having one person act as "Stability Czar" for a pre-approval inspection is commended. Such an individual should be well prepared to respond intelligently to any general question on stability, to identify the location of required data, and to introduce the investigator(s) to the appropriate specialists who can respond in detail to specific technical questions. If no such function exists, it is obviously especially important to give consideration to the coordination of responses to questions concerning stability during the inspection.

D. Conflicting Responses from Different Company Employees

The procedures used by FDA investigators during inspections have been perceived by a number of observers as having changed radically in some districts in recent years. Previously, it seemed to be relatively uncommon for FDA investigators to ask questions of basic-level personnel. Questions were normally directed largely, if not exclusively, to supervisors. Today, perhaps as a result of the generic drug scandal, it seems to be much more common for questions to be addressed to a variety of personnel. Thus, it is important that all employees be clearly instructed on how to respond to questions that an FDA investigator may ask them. The two Golden Rules are (1) always tell the truth; and (2) if you do not know the answer, say so.

Sometimes, junior-level personnel, perhaps feeling either honored or intimidated by being questioned by an FDA investigator, succumb to an attack of acute diarrhea and spout ill-considered, speculative replies to questions. This must be prevented. There are occasions—particularly when responding to a "why" question—when "I don't know" may well be the best, and most honest, answer.

E. Unusual Statistical Treatment of Data

If the sponsor has used some unusual statistical treatment of data, it is helpful to have available at the time of the pre-approval inspection documentation justifying the use of such methods. Documentations such as the minutes of a meeting held in Rockville, MD, at which this subject was discussed, or standard texts on statistics that explain and legitimize the approach, may be useful.

F. Review of 483s

"It's a wise person who learns from their own mistakes; it is a wiser person who learns from someone else's."

A useful exercise for those responsible for stability testing in a company that is preparing for a pre-approval inspection is a careful perusal of 483s (Notice of Adverse Findings) or court case data. Following are points that have emerged from such a review.

The FDA has made it clear that normalization of stability results is not usually desirable. Thus, plots of percentage of label claim as a function of time should not be normalized so that all batches originate at 100% of label claim. In considering batch-to-batch variability in three or more batches, the FDA is interested in both intercepts and slopes. It has been argued, especially in some European countries, that slope dp/dt, where p is potency, is the value of importance in stability testing and that the intercept of such plots need not be considered as far as stability and shelf life is concerned. This argument has not been accepted by the FDA. If, for some special reason, stability data is normalized, then the documentation of the stability results should clearly identify that normalization has been performed and identify the reason for this action.

A number of 483s have commented adversely on stability samples being subjected to delay before testing. Some FDA investigators have adopted a very hard line position in this matter. Thus, if a stability sample is scheduled to be tested on January 6, they have expected that it will be tested on that date—not on January 7 or later. Although this position may well seem to be unrealistically extreme, sponsors should be aware of this potential problem. The answer may lie in documenting in the NDA, ANDA, or other marketing submission document, and the use of the constant date stability testing schedule as described by Carstensen and Rhodes [22].

The calibration, validation, and maintenance of stability chambers have been commented on by several FDA investigators. For example:

> There was no written SOP covering the calibration of the accelerated stability chamber which is used to store the stability samples. In addition, there is no calibration record for this chamber prior to . . .

and

> . . . Failure to have calibrated . . . accelerated chambers temperature monitoring apparatuses to an NBS traceable thermometer. Chamber humidity monitoring device was last calibrated on . . . there is no record maintained documenting this calibration.

In general, temperature control to ±2°C within stability chambers presents no great technical problems, provided that the chamber is not overloaded so that free air flow is restricted. However, if the storage cabinet is overpacked with samples, local, hot, or cold spots can readily develop. The control of RH to ±5% does offer a greater challenge. In selecting stability chambers, the control of RH humidity should be given rigorous attention.

Concern has also been expressed by FDA investigators about the fact that when there were problems in the control of the environment in stability rooms, such problems were not adequately investigated:

> The firm's stability rooms did not provide isolated conditions and/or adequate controls for temperature and relative humidity of drug products placed on stability at room temperature/relative humidity charts for the period . . . revealed that several discrepancies/deficiencies were neither detected nor investigated by Quality Assurance management to assure that stability samples were maintained within the firm's limits.

and

> The firm had no SOP assigning responsibilities for the continuous surveillance and monitoring of temperature and relative humidity in the stability sample areas to assure that retain and stability samples were maintained within the established limits.

and

> Personnel access to the stability area is not restricted or traceable.

and

> . . . The firm lacks adequate control over monitoring of the . . . chamber used to store samples for accelerated stability studies in that:

a. there is no procedure requiring the review, evaluation, and sign-off of recording charts for this chamber;

b. there is no procedure or documentation for calibration of the measurement equipment in this chamber;

c. there are several instances where the charts are missing or incomplete during . . . and . . . which reflects equipment malfunction or breakdown. For example, there are no charts for the period from . . . through . . . ;

d. the review of the T-RH Charts for the period . . . revealed that the RH consistently exceeded the . . . specified in the firm's accelerated stability study procedure.

Attention has also been directed by FDA investigators to computer use in stability studies:

There is no procedure for the operation and control over the computer software used for input/output of stability data and monitoring of the firm's stability studies.

Record keeping and training have also been commented on:

. . . failure to maintain complete records of all stability testing. Records that were maintained lacked adequate information or signature of a second person showing review and acceptance of the results and that they comply with the established standards.

. . . The responsible laboratory employee did not appear to have the proper education, training, and experience to perform the assigned functions and provide assurance that the results are accurate.

As previously indicated, any suggestion of possibly fraudulent changes in records are likely to be a major problem:

. . . record keeping procedures are inadequate. For example, obliteration of information was noted in various documents without identification of the person blanking out the information. . . . record entries are not made as procedures occur. . . . labeling inventory control records are not completed.

When there is any problem data, a formal investigation should be completed and a comprehensive report issued:

. . . When dosage form content uniformity or dissolution testing through all stages result in out-of-specification results, and is deemed as not an equipment, analyst, nor sample error, the firm's SOP (Analytical Testing and Retesting for Chemical Potency Assays) allows for a determination of "inconclusive" cause, and permits retesting, without formal investigation.

. . . The SOP's for testing/retesting do not show procedures to be used when out-of-specification results are found by an outside contract laboratory.

... When an investigation of an out-of-specification result leads to a lab-related issue, there is no provision in the SOP's for extending the investigation to determine if other lots or other product analyses could have been likewise affected by the equipment or analyst.

... for . . . Oral Suspension the validation study does not address additional release specifications potentially related to product handling and storage, such as moisture determination.

The validation of analytical methods used in stability testing has been a subject of concern:

... The firm failed to meet acceptable chromatographic system suitability in the stability assays performed on the ANDA submission batches, in that the standards were run from one to three days prior to those of the samples.

... The chromatograms in the . . . stability assay of . . . contains an additional peak eluting at about nine minutes. The firm failed to adequately investigate and determine the cause of the additional peak, particularly since the problem only occurred in the 60 ml . . . sample bottles, and that the peak was not present in the surrounding initial and . . . test samples.

Computerization of stability data is common, however, if the process is not fully validated. Adverse comment from FDA investigators is likely:

... There is no documented installation configuration qualification for the Stability System Scientific Software used for stability program documentation, monitoring and scheduling. Reportedly, 100% of the active stability projects have been entered and the system is presently used for the Master Stability Record. A non-finalized written validation plan was made available, but the hardware and software installation qualification will be done later, although the system is already being used.

... Lack of a written procedure establishing the steps for inactivating (closing) stability projects in the Stability System Scientific Software. A procedure was drafted on . . . following the observation but lacks the criteria for closing projects and a detailed explanation for documenting the reasons for these activities. At the present time, there is no system that contains organized documentation which clearly provides the reasons for closing or deleting stability projects.

... Failure to maintain a backup log and provide appropriate traceability controls for the Stability Scientific System data separate from the electronic log that is automatically generated for unattended backup to ensure a record is kept in the event of system failure and the electronic log cannot be assessed.

VIII. CONCLUSION

Stability testing is often a critical element in a pre-approval inspection. Thoughtful, objective preparation before the inspection and cooperative coordination during the inspection can greatly reduce and possibly even eliminate problems.

ACKNOWLEDGMENTS

Although the author has been privileged to gain insights into stability testing by his association with numerous pharmaceutical companies, the USP, the FDA, and many individual scientists and regulators, the views expressed in this chapter are not represented as reflecting the views of anyone other than the author.

The author thanks Dr. Jens Carstensen, Dr. S. Valvani, Dr. D. Hong, and Mr. D. Dean for providing him with ideas and facts that have assisted him in writing this chapter.

REFERENCES

1. *FDA Guidelines for Submitting Documentation for the Stability of Human Drugs and Biologics*, February 1987.
2. International Conference on Harmonization (ICH) Harmonized Tripartite Guideline, *Stability Testing on New Drug Substances and Products*, 1993.
3. J. T. Carstensen, *Drug Stability: Principles and Practices*, Second Edition, Marcel Dekker, 1995.
4. *FDA Compliance Program Manual Guide*, August 15, 1994.
5. *FDA Proposed Amendment to CGMP Requirement*, 21 CFR, Parts 210 and 211, May 3, 1996.
6. Federal Register, March 1, 1995, pp. 1120–1126.
7. *Reviewer Guidance—Validation of Chromatographic Methods*, CEDER, November 1994.
8. *FDA Guideline for Submitting Samples and Analytical Data for Methods Validation*, 1987.
9. Federal Register, International Conference on Harmonization, *Guideline on Validation of Analytical Procedure*, March 1, 1995, March 7, 1996.
10. USP 23, 1995, p. 1776, *et seq.*
11. FDA Reviewer Guidance, *Validation of Chromatographic Methods*, November 1994.
12. *Acceptable Methods*, Health Protection Board, Health Welfare Canada, 1994.
13. R. D. C. Jones, B. A. Matthews, C. T. Rhodes, *J. Pharm. Sci.* 59:518–523 (1970).
14. L. J. Leeson, *Dissolution Technologies* 4:5–9 (1997).

15. S. Bolton, *Pharmaceutical Stability: Practical and Clinical Applications*, Second Edition, New York, Marcel Dekker, 1992.
16. *International Pharmaceutical Product Registration*, A. C. Cartright, B. R. Matthews, eds. Ellis Horwood, 1994.
17. H. L. Avalone, *Pharm. Eng.* 10:38–41 (1990).
18. K. M. Morisseau, C. T. Rhodes, *Drug Dev. Ind. Pharm.* 21:1071–1090 (1995).
19. P. Nakagaki, AAPS Las Vegan Meeting, 1990.
20. P. Helbae, *Drug Information J.* 26:629–634 (1992).
21. C. T. Rhodes, *Clin. Res. Drug Reg. Affairs* 10:65–69 (1993).
22. J. T. Carstensen, C. T. Rhodes, *Clin. Res. Drug Reg. Affairs* 10:177–185 (1993).

5

Consequences of Failing a Pre-Approval Inspection

Arthur N. Levine
Arnold & Porter, Washington, D.C.

I. INTRODUCTION

Failing a Food and Drug Administration (FDA) pre-approval inspection can have serious consequences for the New Drug Application (NDA) or supplement that is the subject of the inspection and on other drugs manufactured by the NDA applicant. The most direct consequences are delay in obtaining FDA approval, the need for the company to repeat or revalidate study data, and, where the failure is due to deficiencies in current good manufacturing practices (GMPs), the need for the company to modify manufacturing or quality assurance procedures. These direct consequences result from the fact that the FDA will not approve an NDA or NDA supplement on the basis of data that have serious unexplained inconsistencies or discrepancies, nor will the FDA approve an application if there are significant GMP deficiencies at the facility in which the drug will be manufactured.

This chapter reviews the direct consequences of failing a pre-approval inspection and identifies and discusses the less direct but very real additional consequences that may confront a company.

In November 1997, Congress passed the Food and Drug Administration Modernization Act of 1997 (Modernization Act). Most provisions of the Act became effective in February 1998. Two provisions of the new legislation could affect the consequences of failing a pre-approval inspection. Section 119 of the Modernization Act amends the new drug provisions of the federal Food, Drug,

119

and Cosmetic Act to provide that no action by the NDA reviewing division "may be delayed because of the unavailability of information from or because of action by field personnel" unless the reviewing division determines that "a delay is necessary to assure the marketing of a safe and effective drug" [21 U.S.C. § 355(b)(4)(F), as amended]. This provision suggests that review personnel may overrule the concerns and objections by FDA district office personnel regarding the impact on NDA approval of GMP and other deficiencies observed during a pre-approval inspection. It also suggests that the inability of a district office to perform a scheduled pre-approval inspection—resulting in "unavailability of information"—may be an inadequate basis for delaying approval of an NDA if the reviewing division is otherwise satisfied and inclined to proceed.

In addition, the Modernization Act further amends the new drug provisions by authorizing written decisions by the NDA reviewing division to memorialize agreements with an NDA applicant about the design and size of clinical trials intended to demonstrate safety and effectiveness. As amended, the new drug provisions now provide that these written decisions "shall be binding upon, and may not directly or indirectly be changed by, the field or compliance division personnel unless such field or compliance division personnel demonstrate to the reviewing division why such decision should be modified" [21 U.S.C. § 355(b)(4)(E), as amended]. This provision suggests that where data developed to support an NDA are the result of procedures approved in a written decision by the NDA reviewing division, FDA district investigators will have a burden of persuading the reviewing division that the procedures are inadequate to generate reliable data in support of an NDA approval decision and should be modified.

These provisions of the Modernization Act do not appear to be designed to accomplish a fundamental alteration in the pre-approval inspection process. Moreover, as a practical matter, reviewing divisions can be expected to give substantial weight to the concerns and objections raised by FDA field personnel respecting the impact of pre-approval inspection deficiencies on the safety and efficacy of a drug. It is likely that significant GMP deviations will be found by NDA reviewing division personnel as justifying a delay in NDA approval. Field personnel will remind NDA reviewers that the statutory purpose of the GMPs is to assure that a drug is safe and has the quality that it purports to have [21 U.S.C. § 351(a)(2)(B)]. These practical accommodations notwithstanding, the new provisions do, however, seem to alter the balance of authority within the agency to resolve GMP and data integrity issues by giving the reviewing division a more preeminent role in resolving these issues.

At the time of this publication, the FDA had not revised its pre-approval inspection program or related policies described in this chapter in response to the Modernization Act. It is likely that the impetus for change will come when individual companies are confronted with concerns and objections raised by field personnel. These companies will rely on the Modernization Act amendments in arguing against delay in approval of their applications.

II. FACTORS THAT DETERMINE WHAT THE CONSEQUENCES MAY BE

The nature and extent of the consequences of failing an NDA pre-approval inspection depend on three elements: (1) the reason for failure; (2) whether the reason affects only the pending NDA that is the subject of the inspection; and (3) the specific recommendation and broader enforcement philosophy of the FDA District Office conducting or participating in the pre-approval inspection.

A. The Reason for Failure

The FDA's pre-approval inspection program guidance identifies five reasons why a company might fail a pre-approval inspection: (1) significant deviations from the GMP regulations, including pre-approval batches not being made in conformance with GMPs; (2) deviation from other "application commitments"; (3) inconsistencies or discrepancies "raising significant questions about the validity of records"; (4) failure to report adverse findings or test data without adequate justification; and (5) suspicion of fraud, such as creation of documents known to contain false information.

Significant GMP deviations, questions about the validity of records, and suspicion of fraud are the kinds of reasons for failure that can more easily lead to consequences beyond the application that is the subject of the pre-approval inspection. When the inspection deficiencies are limited to the pending NDA, the consequences will also be limited to delaying approval.

B. Tainting Other Data or Processes

When deficiencies relating to the drug that is the subject of the pre-approval inspection directly implicate other pending NDAs or supplements, or when there are sufficient parallels between the deficiencies observed during the pre-approval inspection and the procedures and controls applicable to the company's marketed products, the pre-approval inspection may spill over to the company's other products. Common elements between the drug that is the subject of the pre-approval inspection and other drugs manufactured by the company provide pathways for broader regulatory consequences.

These common elements may include the use of the same raw materials or components, the use of the same equipment (particularly sterilization equipment), application of the same manufacturing procedures (particularly when those procedures are critical to determining significant quality characteristics of the drugs), or reliance on the same validation data. The participation of a particular employee, supervisor, or manager may also be a common element linking concerns about the pre-approval drug to other drugs manufactured by the applicant. When the FDA discovers what it believes is fraud in the records applicable to one study, its inspectional focus may be expanded to include pivotal studies for approved drugs performed by the same clinical investigator, studies subject to review by the same company monitor or generated by the same group or division within the company.

The more focused the deficiencies are to the application that is the subject of pre-approval inspection, the more circumscribed the consequences. The more potentially applicable the deficiencies are to the company's other products, the greater the possibility for consequences affecting the company's other products.

C. The Role of the FDA District Office

The views of the FDA District Office conducting or participating in the pre-approval inspection can, and often will, significantly influence the consequences of the inspection, including the possible spillover to other drug products manufactured by the company.

However, the ability of the District Office to influence NDA reviewing division personnel, and to effectuate any district concerns or objections arising out of a pre-approval inspection, appear to have been undercut by the amendments to the new drug provisions provided by the Modernization Act that give the reviewing division the preeminent role in assessing the need for any delay in an NDA review based on any action by field personnel. A recommendation from the District Office that FDA withhold drug approval is likely to face a more searching assessment by the NDA reviewing division. A loss of equal status with the reviewing division is, however, unlikely to discourage district personnel from pursuing other regulatory consequences arising from the discovery of GMP-deficient practices or unreliable data available under the federal Food, Drug, and Cosmetic Act, as described in this chapter.

The District Office will ordinarily be the first to evaluate the results of the pre-approval inspection [1].

In addition, in nearly all circumstances, it is the responsibility of the District Office to recommend a regulatory response to the deficiencies observed during any FDA inspection. Districts may be more or less inclined to pursue a wider, more encompassing response to inspectional deviations depending on the enforcement philosophy of the District Director or the Director of the Compliance

Branch. Similarly, each District Office Inspections Branch may be more or less capable of identifying and documenting evidence of the kind of deficiencies suggesting deviations, discrepancies, or fraud extending beyond the application that is the subject of a pre-approval inspection. In other words, both the enforcement orientation and the technical skill of district personnel can affect the extent to which the consequences of failing a pre-approval inspection remain limited and focused or are widened and expanded. Moreover, at any point in time, the available resources of the district to thoroughly investigate apparent deviations, inconsistencies, or discrepancies may vary.

The role of District Offices in pre-approval inspections brings an FDA's "field" perspective into the NDA approval process. While Center for Drug Evaluation and Review (CDER) medical reviewers tend to focus on an application, FDA District Offices tend to focus on companies and their facilities, processes, and systems. CDER medical reviewers are responsible for evaluating the data submitted. They are not charged with determining why a company has failed to provide the necessary data as prescribed in the NDA regulations. District investigators are trained to look for connections and patterns to discover whether deficiencies in the conditions under which one drug is made also exist in the conditions under which other drugs are made by the same company in the same facility. In addition, a district's perspective is remedial; district compliance officials expect that deficient conditions will be fixed, not merely explained.

Given these variables—the reason for the failure, the apparent or possible relationship between the pending application and other products in the company's product line, and the approach of the District Office—the consequences of failing a pre-approval inspection can be either narrow or broad.

III. THE CONSEQUENCES OF FAILING A PRE-APPROVAL INSPECTION ON THE DRUG THAT IS THE SUBJECT OF THE APPLICATION

A. Delay in Product Approval

The most immediate consequence of failing a pre-approval inspection is a delay in FDA approval of the application or supplement. FDA District Offices recommend withholding approval of approximately 30% of the pending NDA applications for which pre-approval inspections have been conducted.

The extent of a change in the relationship between NDA reviewing divisions and FDA district offices under the amendments to the new drug provisions enacted as part of the Modernization Act is yet to be fully determined. The

District Office's co-equal status appears, however, to have been Congressionally undermined.

The delay is usually not limited to FDA reconsideration of the data in the application and the inspectional findings. More often, to resolve questions raised during the pre-approval inspection, the FDA will request additional data to reach a level of assurance that any deviations, inconsistencies, or discrepancies have been explained or overcome. This may include the FDA requiring that equipment or process validations be repeated, that pilot batches be rerun, that manufacturing procedures be revised, or that tests on active ingredients or finished drugs be repeated. If the FDA concludes that a significant or pivotal study (or laboratory data) supporting the pending application is not reliable, the study will have to be repeated.

If approval is withheld for a long time or if it becomes apparent that the FDA will not approve an application, many companies will withdraw the application rather than experience an outright FDA refusal to approve.

B. Increased FDA Investigations

Failing an initial pre-approval inspection may result in a reinspection to verify the new data, revised procedures, or repeated testing. While the reinspection will be initially focused on the concerns that prevented the District Office from endorsing the NDA approval, a district investigator is never precluded from documenting a significant GMP deviation or investigating an appearance of fraud that the investigator may observe. No FDA inspection is completely predictable, and all require the careful attention and dedicated resources of the company.

Another consequence of failing a pre-approval inspection due to inconsistencies or discrepancies in the study data may be an FDA inspection of one or more clinical investigator sites. Such visits usually focus on comparing the data in the NDA submission, the data in the company's records, and the original data collected by the clinical investigator.

The FDA increased the number of on-site clinical inspections significantly during the mid-1990s. More significantly, the FDA data show that the Agency found what it believed were deviations from requirements for conducting clinical trials in more than three quarters of those inspections and in more than three quarters of its inspections at institutional review boards. The problems that the FDA discovers most frequently are deficiencies in obtaining informed consent, nonadherence to protocols, inaccurate or inadequate records, or failing to adequately monitor drug accountability.

While the principal sanction imposed by the FDA for significant deficiencies in clinical investigations is assessed against the investigator, who can be declared ineligible to receive investigational drugs or may be restricted in the kind of research that he or she may conduct, these deficiencies can also haunt the sponsor. Not only are sponsors generally accountable for using appropriate clinical investigators [2], the FDA may reject clinical studies used to support an NDA if the investigator is unqualified or if deviations from the FDA's investigational new drug (IND) requirements or the test protocol are significant. Significant deficiencies in pivotal studies usually preclude approval until reliable data can be generated.

These consequences, although never desirable, are circumscribed and usually involve only a delay in the approval. Moreover, while the company may have to validate data, generate new data, or revise its manufacturing processes, these requirements parallel what the company has already done in preparing the NDA. However, should the FDA suspect fraud or a lack of authenticity in documents supporting the NDA, it may invoke its Applications Integrity Policy (initially known as the Fraud Policy). This significantly ups the ante.

C. The Applications Integrity Policy

Under the FDA's Applications Integrity Policy, if the Agency concludes that data in a pending application are unreliable, it will "defer substantive scientific review of the application" until questions regarding reliability of the data have been resolved and the company has satisfied the FDA that the application, and the data supporting it, are valid and authentic. The policy on fraud, untrue statements of material facts, bribery, and illegal gratuities was published in the *Federal Register* on September 10, 1991 [3].

The Applications Integrity Policy can be invoked without concrete evidence of fraud; it may be invoked because of a suspicion of fraud. Although the policy is supposed to be applied "only when there is a pattern of practice of wrongful conduct that raises a significant question regarding the reliability of data in an application," the FDA has announced that data "may be unreliable due to sloppiness or inadvertent errors." Thus, simple errors in the recording of data may be adequate to call the reliability of the data into question and thus provide the basis for the FDA invoking the Applications Integrity Policy. While the power to invoke the Applications Integrity Policy rests with the Center, a forceful presentation for invoking the policy by the District Office conducting the pre-approval inspection will be given great weight.

Once the policy is invoked, a company must: (1) conduct its own internal review to identify any wrongful conduct or discrepancies and provide the results of the review to the FDA; (2) identify for the FDA all individuals who "were or may have been associated with wrongful acts," and (3) remove these individuals from any substantive authority in the company on matters under the FDA's jurisdiction (thus, as part of a company's compliance with the Applications

Integrity Policy, it may be required, in effect, to debar some of its own employees). A company must also cooperate fully with the FDA and other federal investigation officials who may be investigating the cause, scope, and effects of any wrongdoing. Obviously, the internal review and the other corrective measures required of companies are time consuming and extremely disruptive, even when focused on the particular application that was the subject matter of the pre-approval inspection.

For example, according to the FDA's *Points to Consider for Internal Reviews and Corrective Action Operating Plans*, a company's internal review should include an analysis of the problems identified by the FDA in its notice to the applicant, a specific audit plan, the audits themselves, and submission of the audit reports to the FDA. The Agency has encouraged companies to use an outside consultant or team of consultants to conduct their audit and to submit the audit plan for FDA review before implementation. According to the FDA, the scope of the audit plan should "identify all personnel to be interviewed; the functions, specific activities and products that may be affected; and all associated data, records, samples, specimens and other documentations that could reveal information about the wrongful acts" [4].

After the company conducts its own audit and provides the FDA with all of the information it has discovered, the Agency may undertake its own audit, called a "validity assessment," to verify that the company's internal audit has been completed satisfactorily and that the corrective action plan is implemented and operational. (The FDA has specifically advised some companies that it will not accept a company's internal audit without further Agency review.) In addition, as part of its validity assessment, the FDA is free to independently pursue any evidence of fraud that becomes known to it, either as the result of the company's internal audit or the FDA's own investigation. The FDA will not release a company and its pending application from the policy until the FDA has conducted its validity assessment to the extent and depth that it deems appropriate.

The FDA takes the position that invoking the Applications Integrity Policy does not, in itself, prevent the FDA's ultimate approval of the application. Thus, the FDA has concluded that companies do not have a right to a hearing to challenge their being subjected to the policy. However, being subjected to the policy can have a substantial impact on a company, particularly when the FDA defers review of applications supported by data for which it has no direct evidence of fraud. In these circumstances, judicial challenge to the policy may be successful.

The existence of the Applications Integrity Policy has provided the FDA with significant leverage in "encouraging" companies to withdraw NDAs until questions concerning the validity or authenticity of the data can be resolved.

As long as a company is operating under the policy, any affected application will be delayed. Satisfaction of the terms of the policy are rarely achieved overnight. For example, in September 1994, Fujisawa USA, Inc. issued a news release announcing that the FDA had notified it that the company was no longer subject to the Agency's Applications Integrity Policy. According to the release, the policy was invoked by the FDA in March 1992, two and a half years earlier. The Applications Integrity Policy delayed for 18 months the FDA review of four abbreviated NDAs (ANDAs) submitted by Royce Laboratories. A number of manufacturers of generic drugs have been subjected to the Applications Integrity Policy, resulting in withdrawal of applications and lengthy delays in FDA review of numerous pending applications.

D. Debarment

The Generic Drug Enforcement Act of 1992 gave the FDA authority to administratively debar individuals who participated in or countenanced fraud in the development of any drug. Many elements of the FDA's debarment power are limited to ANDAs. However, an individual who has been debarred may not provide services in any capacity to any company that has an approved or pending NDA or ANDA [5]. When a company submits an NDA or ANDA to the FDA for review and approval, it must certify to the Agency that it did not use the services of any debarred individual in developing or submitting the application [6]. A company may be assessed a civil penalty of up to $1 million for knowingly using the services of a debarred individual [7]. A debarred individual may be ordered to pay a civil penalty of up to $250,000 for providing services to any company with a pending application.

An individual can be debarred if he or she has been convicted of a felony under federal law for conduct relating to the development or approval of any drug subject to FDA approval. An individual may also be debarred for having engaged in criminal conduct "relating to the regulation" of any FDA-approved drug [8].

An individual may be debarred if he or she "materially participated" in any conduct that was the basis of a conviction, even if the individual was not himself or herself convicted, if the FDA has reason to believe that the individual may violate FDA requirements concerning drugs [9]. The FDA may also debar an officer, director, or other "high managerial agent" of a company if that person knew of conduct by either superiors or subordinates that resulted in a felony conviction and subsequent debarment of one or more of these superiors or subordinates and that person did not report the misconduct to the FDA or failed to take other action to prevent it. The basis for debarment may be imposed only if the "high managerial agent" knew about the misconduct or avoided learning about it.

An individual may be debarred only after an opportunity for a hearing before the FDA on disputed issues of material fact [10]. However, the opportunity to a hearing is not the same as a right to a hearing. The FDA can deny a request for a hearing if undisputed issues of material fact are adequate to support the debarment.

The names of debarred individuals are published in the *Federal Register* and the FDA maintains a list of them that is publicly available [11]. Approximately 30 individuals have been debarred by the FDA since the law became effective.

As is apparent, information that companies have developed during an internal audit under the Applications Integrity Policy parallels the information that would support the debarment of individuals in the company, thus precluding them, in effect, from employment in the pharmaceutical industry. The possibility that adherence to the Applications Integrity Policy could generate data supporting debarment is furthered by the requirement that a company identify to the FDA all persons who may have been associated with any wrongdoing. Of course, if a company's internal audit did not disclose information that would support a debarment, the FDA's own "validity assessment" could yield such information independently.

E. Criminal Investigation

Delaying NDA approval, demanding further data, invoking the Applications Integrity Policy, or debarring company officials are all administrative sanctions that the FDA can invoke on its own as a consequence of a company failing a pre-approval inspection. The FDA need not obtain the approval of the Justice Department or any other federal law enforcement agency to impose these sanctions. However, serious discrepancies regarding the validity or authenticity of documents submitted to the FDA, intentional fraud, or knowing concealment of material facts from the Agency, may well constitute violations of federal criminal law. Evidence of such illegal conduct may be forwarded by the FDA to the Justice Department for criminal investigation and, ultimately, prosecution. Moreover, in many circumstances, imposition of FDA administrative sanctions does not preclude the Department of Justice from prosecuting the same conduct criminally.

1. The FDA's Office of Criminal Investigations

At any time during an investigation of suspected fraud, the FDA can turn to its Office of Criminal Investigations (OCI), which consists of approximately 120 specially trained criminal investigators located in six offices throughout the United States. The OCI focuses its investigative efforts on fraud and the submission of false information to the FDA [12]. OCI investigators are authorized to carry firearms, and most have extensive experience in criminal investigations. The FDA has exempted from disclosure to the public written agreements and Memoranda of Understanding between the OCI and other departments, agencies, and organizations because those "could reveal confidential investigative techniques or disclose guidelines for investigations that may interfere with law enforcement" [13].

Like other FDA investigators, OCI investigators carry FDA credentials that they are required to present at the beginning of an inspection or when joining an ongoing inspection [14]. However, while FDA district investigators carry Agency credentials designated 200A or 200B, OCI investigators carry 200D or 200E credentials. Thus, a company can often determine whether the FDA has decided to use its OCI investigators, a decision that usually signals a preliminary FDA assessment that evidence of criminally fraudulent activity may exist.

2. The Justice Department's Office of Consumer Litigation

Whether the FDA gathers evidence of criminal fraud through its district investigators or through its OCI investigators, that information will ordinarily be forwarded to the Office of Consumer Litigation (OCL), a part of the Justice Department that is principally responsible for coordinating both criminal prosecutions and civil injunction and seizure actions for violations of the Federal Food, Drug, and Cosmetic Act.

Ordinarily, the OCL will either direct the investigation and be actively involved in any criminal prosecution that may result or will ask that one of the 96 U.S. Attorney's Office handle the case. The OCL has taken the leading role in the investigation and presentation of nearly all of the intentional violations involving the FDA for more than 20 years. Its experience, and the expertise of attorneys in the FDA's Chief Counsel's office, present a formidable obstacle to companies and individuals seeking to avoid prosecution once the FDA has made a referral.

In addition, the U.S. Attorney's Office in Baltimore, Maryland, has established a special prosecution staff that evolved from its leading role in prosecuting fraud in the generic drug industry. Working with the FDA's investigators, it will often take an active role in pursuing evidence of fraud involving FDA-regulated drugs.

3. The Justice Department's Health Care Fraud Office

Preliminary information developed by the FDA concerning fraud in the NDA may be included within the purview of the Deputy to the Attorney General for health care fraud, for investigational support, and coordination under the Justice Department's health care fraud initiative. Reflecting that Department's "renewed commitment to health-care fraud and enforcement," the number of cases prosecuted under this program increased significantly during the mid-1990s and criminal investigations for "health care fraud" increased more than threefold during that time. The Deputy in charge of the health care fraud program reports that more than 600 Federal Bureau of Investigation (FBI) agents have been assigned to health care fraud cases. The Department has also developed a database of United States Attorney's Offices and Justice Department attorneys with health care fraud expertise to share with law enforcement agencies, including the FDA [15].

The Justice Department includes within the program the prosecution of C. R. Bard, Inc., for defrauding the FDA. The company agreed to pay a $30 million fine and an additional $30 million in civil claims. In March 1996, the Justice Department announced that Circa Pharmaceuticals agreed to pay a $2.7 million fine to resolve allegations that it sold untested generic drugs to the U.S. government and government-funded programs from 1986 through March 1991. The agreement reportedly settles Circa's civil liability under the False Claims Act and common law and brings to $13.7 million the total fines paid by Circa and its predecessor, Bolar.

4. Criminal Investigation

The most significant consequence of the FDA referring information concerning possible fraud to the Justice Department for further investigation is the scope of that Department's criminal investigative powers. For example, although the FDA has no general subpoena power, investigative grand juries, working at the direction of Assistant U.S. Attorneys or Justice Department Attorneys, can issue subpoenas to compel the production of evidence and testimony that may be necessary to develop criminal charges. In addition, only Assistant U.S. Attorneys or other Justice Department attorneys may obtain from a United States judge or magistrate a criminal search warrant to obtain evidence of violations of law. Similarly, only Justice Department lawyers can seek authorization to engage in sophisticated electronic surveillance. Finally, Assistant U.S. Attorneys and other Justice Department lawyers can offer immunity from prosecution and enter into favorable plea bargains with persons who have valuable information to obtain their cooperation in building cases against other targets.

The existence of these investigative techniques significantly increases the exposure of companies and individuals to criminal prosecution based on fraud associated with NDA submissions. Even if criminal charges are never brought, criminal investigations are enormously disruptive to a company and have a significant adverse effect on employee morale. If the existence of a grand jury investigation is leaked, the consequences can be expected to attract stock market analysts, the media, shareholder groups, product liability lawyers, and many others.

Moreover, whether the FDA invokes the Application Integrity Policy or not, it will not review a pending NDA that is the subject of a criminal investigation predicated on a suspicion of fraud or a lack of authenticity of records in the application.

IV. CONSEQUENCES OF FAILING A PRE-APPROVAL INSPECTION ON DRUGS THAT ARE NOT THE SUBJECT OF THE INSPECTION

Apart from adverse consequences related directly to the drug that is the subject of the pre-approval inspection, there may be consequences for other products of the company, both those being marketed and those for which an NDA or supplement is pending before the FDA. As described in Section II of this chapter, the spillover from the drug that is the subject of the pre-approval inspection to other products can be narrow or broad, depending on the relationship between deviations, inconsistencies, discrepancies, or suspicions of fraud associated with the NDA that is the subject of the pre-approval inspection, and the data, processes, or key personnel working on the company's other products.

A. Increased FDA Inspections

The most likely circumstances for potential spillover is the FDA's discovery of significant GMP deviations during the pre-approval inspection. If the FDA identifies what it believes are significant GMP deviations in the production (of pilot batches) of the drug offered for approval, or in the record keeping or other processes associated with that drug, that are common to other drugs that the company manufactures, the Agency may expand the scope of its investigation. If the FDA discovers what it believes are significant discrepancies in records that call into question their authenticity or raise the suspicion of fraud with respect to the drug subject to the NDA pre-approval inspection, it is likely that the FDA will expand the scope of its investigation. The expanded investigation will focus on the significant GMP processes, procedures and systems, and pivotal data associated with the other drugs.

Once the FDA moves beyond the focused parameters of the pre-approval inspection, a broader range of the company's manufacturing processes are exposed to scrutiny and criticism. Moreover, because the inspection has been expanded due to the FDA investigator's belief that there are deficiencies associated with the pending NDA drug, the expanded investigation begins with a heightened level of apprehension or concern. This, in subtle but very real ways, generally results in a more searching FDA review. Should an FDA investigator suspect fraud, the investigator may act as if the burden of demonstrating the reliability of the data rests with the company rather than the burden being on the FDA investigator to discover and document inconsistencies in the data.

If the reason for the expanded inspection is significant GMP deficiencies, a number of FDA regulatory consequences may result. GMP deficiencies are the leading reason for failures in pre-approval inspections. They are also the leading cause for the issuance of FDA warning letters, the most frequently referenced basis for an allegation of adulteration resulting in a product recall or an FDA seizure, and the deficiency most likely to lead to an FDA recommendation for injunction.

B. Products Not Yet Marketed

1. Delay in Product Approval

The FDA will not approve any pending NDAs or supplements if it believes that there are significant GMP deficiencies at the facility where the drugs would be manufactured. Thus, failing a pre-approval inspection for a particular drug due to systemic and serious GMP deviations may result in the FDA declining to approve other applications until the deficiencies applicable to the manufacture of the other drugs are corrected.

The FDA has maintained a computerized tracking system, called the Compliance Inspection Tracking System (CIRTS), that monitors inspection results for all FDA inspections. The CIRTS contains information on a company's compliance history and on its recent inspectional findings. Based on information available under CIRTS, the FDA may put an application on hold until the company can demonstrate that it is in compliance with GMPs. In theory, the FDA should not delay review of a pending application unless the GMP deficiencies are applicable to the manufacture of that particular drug. However, the Agency can often find linkage between products.

2. Impact on Ongoing Research

Failing a pre-approval inspection for a pending NDA can have an adverse effect on drugs undergoing clinical research under an IND exemption, particularly when the IND drug is the same as the pending NDA drug and the IND has been made in the same facility, on the same equipment, under the same manufacturing practices, and by the same company employees as the pending NDA drug. In addition, the IND drug may be supported by some of the same basic safety and toxicology data as the pending NDA drug. Finally, clinical data supporting the IND drug may have been generated by the same clinical investigator or may have been supervised by the same company monitor as the pending NDA drug.

Evidence of GMP deficiencies or deficiencies in preclinical or clinical data discovered during the pre-approval inspection may directly undermine representations in the IND. The FDA can call for the same kinds of revalidation or repetition of data as for the pending NDA. The Agency also may take action to curtail the progress of the IND, including placing a clinical hold on the IND if, for example, a lack of confidence in data on the drug's toxicity should arise.

3. The Applications Integrity Policy

The FDA can invoke the Applications Integrity Policy based on a lack of confidence in the authenticity and reliability of the data in any application. Beginning with suspicions about fraud or irregularities in data in the NDA that is the subject of the pre-approval inspection, the zone of FDA suspicion may extend to pending applications and supplements submitted by a company during a particular time period; to those generated by a particular division of a company or subject to the supervision of a particular supervisor or official; or to applications supported by data by a particular outside contract laboratory, or subject to control by a company's clinical investigations monitor. In each case, the FDA will have made a preliminary conclusion that it no longer has confidence in the reliability of the data generated by that part of the company's operations that appear to be responsible for the suspect data.

The FDA has made clear that it may invoke its Applications Integrity Policy against pending applications and supplements other than those in which there is direct evidence of fraud:

> [A] policy limiting validity assessments and deferral of substantive scientific review to applications in which the Agency has actually discovered evidence of fraud or untrue statements would be inadequate. . . . A validity assessment will ordinarily be triggered by an Agency determination that evidence of wrongful acts has raised questions about the reliability of data in an application or applications.

The nature of the assessment and the determination of which applications are affected will depend on the facts of the particular case. Thus, the validity assessment process may be narrowly focused on one or a few applications when, for example, the Agency concludes that one individual is wholly responsible for wrongful acts and that the misconduct could have affected only a few identified applications. On the other hand, the validity assessment process may be extensive if the FDA believes that the scope of the wrongful act may be broader:

> FDA does not agree that validity assessment should necessarily be limited to applications for which there is a direct relationship between the wrongful acts and the questioned data.

When the FDA notifies a company that the Applications Integrity Policy is being invoked on a broad basis, it will expect that the company's internal audit will be equally broad in its design and scope. Similarly, the breadth and depth of the company's corrective measures will need to parallel the FDA's perception of the scope of the suspected fraud. Indeed, the FDA has advised companies that in implementing corrective actions "applicants may need to revise manufacturing practices, hiring practices, training procedures and other areas of operations to ensure reliability of data."

4. Criminal Investigation

The FDA's suspicions concerning the authenticity and reliability of NDA data, or its suspicions of the existence of fraud in a company's documents associated with pending applications and supplements for drugs other than those that were the focus of the pre-approval inspection, can also lead to a criminal investigation. In fact, even if company documents are not submitted to the FDA, they may be within the FDA's jurisdiction because they may influence an FDA decision or are subject to inspection by the FDA. Accordingly, such documents can be the basis of federal criminal violation under 18 U.S.C. § 1001. Therefore, even though a product is not yet marketed, intentional fraud associated with that product may provide the basis for criminal prosecution.

A conviction for violating 18 U.S.C. § 1001 may, in turn, be the basis for debarring an individual, although conviction of a crime is not a necessary prerequisite for debarment in some circumstances.

C. Marketed Products

Significant GMP deficiencies first identified during a pre-approval inspection can result in a host of FDA regulatory actions adversely affecting other drugs already approved for marketing.

1. Warning Letters

A company may receive a warning letter from the FDA identifying GMP deficiencies, or containing Agency allegations regarding data integrity, applicable to one or more of a company's marketed drugs. The warning letter notifies a company of the Agency's expectations that the company should correct the deficiencies identified in the letter. Some warning letters include the FDA's position that the company should retain outside expert consultants to assist in resolving the deficiencies, and the letter may call for certification of compliance by those consultants. The warning letter may also ask that copies of the consultants' reports be submitted to the FDA. Warning letters generally call for companies to respond within 3 weeks (15 working days) of receiving the letter. While a company need not have implemented all of the corrections within that time, the FDA expects that its response will provide reasonably accurate target times for completion.

However, a warning letter is not a private admonition from the FDA. Warning letters are publicly available under the Freedom of Information Act, and many of them are affirmatively put on public display by the FDA in its Docket Management Office. In addition, the pharmaceutical trade press routinely reports on warning letters, and a separate trade publication is devoted exclusively to tracking warning letters. The trade press will publish articles on warning letters if the circumstances—the size or identity of the company receiving the letter, the popularity of the drug affected by the warning letter, the remedial steps demanded by the warning letter—are perceived as newsworthy. The company's response to the FDA is also a publicly available document. The existence of this correspondence in the public domain can attract not only the trade press, but also the media, product liability lawyers, security analysts, competitors, and other people whose interests are served by monitoring the regulatory difficulties of a company or a particular drug.

2. Government Contracts

The FDA sends a copy of its warning letters to federal procurement agencies encouraging them to consider those letters in awarding procurement contracts and in assessing initial procurement acceptability determinations. Thus, failing a pre-approval inspection for one drug can result in the loss of a lucrative federal procurement contract for another.

3. Approved NDAs

If the FDA believes that the deficiencies identified in a pre-approval inspection affect the company's marketed drugs, it can require the company to address those deficiencies in the form of an NDA supplement or a labeling change for one or more of those drugs. In an extreme case, if the FDA believes that the statutory prerequisites have been met, it may issue a notice of opportunity for a hearing announcing its intention to revoke the NDA approval for a drug. A proceeding to revoke an NDA may be based on the FDA's view that approved drugs are not being made in compliance with GMPs, are not made as described in the approved NDA, or that the approval was obtained because the application contained untrue statements of material fact.

4. Recalls and Seizures

If an FDA investigation that started as a pre-approval inspection but spilled over to an investigation of other drugs discloses (1) significant GMP deviations, (2) labeling or promotional practices that cause a drug to be misbranded, or (3) evidence that a particular lot was subpotent, out of specifications, contaminated, or otherwise "adulterated" under the Federal Food, Drug, and Cosmetic Act, the FDA investigator may suggest that the company consider a "voluntary" recall of the particular lot or of several lots of the drug. This suggestion may be in the form of a review of the investigator's findings followed by the question, "What do you intend to do about the drug in the marketplace?" Or an investigator may be more direct, advising a company that the lot or lots are adulterated or misbranded and the investigator intends to recommend enforcement action unless the company agrees to promptly take remedial action. At that point, or within the next few days, the company must advise the FDA of its intentions. If the company decides to initiate a voluntary recall, it may follow (or closely parallel) the FDA's published guidelines for recalls [16].

If an FDA investigator identifies a drug that the investigator believes is adulterated or misbranded and should be removed from commerce, and if the company has not made a commitment to remove it from the market voluntarily, the District Office may forward to FDA headquarters a recommendation that the drug be seized. The likelihood of such a recommendation is the greatest if an FDA investigator collects a sample of the drug, documents a particular condition with photographs or drawings, or collects records showing that the drug or its components have been shipped in interstate commerce.

A seizure may focus on a particular lot of a drug or, if significant GMP deviations are documented that would apply to most or all of the company's drugs, the FDA may forward to the Justice Department a recommendation for a mass seizure. Once accomplished by a Deputy U.S. Marshal, a mass seizure not only removes a substantial quantity of drugs from the company's control (by placing them under the jurisdiction of the court), but can seriously disrupt the company's operations. This is because, in most cases, the drugs will be seized "in place" and thus occupy warehousing, labeling, and even manufacturing space within a facility.

The FDA's objective in a seizure is the condemnation of the drugs followed by either their destruction or reconditioning [17]. Because seizures involve a considerable degree of FDA resources and must be approved by the Justice

Department before they can be filed, the FDA has tended in recent years to pursue administrative remedies, such as issuing warning letters or encouraging companies to conduct recalls. Company recalls and FDA warning letters consume a relatively small amount of FDA resources and put the burden of compliance on the company. Indeed, in each of the past few years, there have been approximately 2500 recalls of FDA-regulated products, approximately 1500 FDA warning letters, and approximately 100 seizures.

5. Injunction

If the FDA believes that the pre-approval inspection for one drug has uncovered serious drug quality or GMP deficiencies associated with one or more of the company's other drugs, the FDA may recommend that the Justice Department file a Complaint for Injunction [18]. Typically, the complaint will seek—either by consent of a company or by court order after a judicial proceeding—that the company be precluded from manufacturing or distributing the drugs until prescribed remedial measures, identified by the FDA, are implemented. A "standard" injunction order will require that the company's compliance be certified by an outside expert and confirmed by an FDA inspection. The particular terms imposed on a company under an injunction usually parallel the circumstances that have led the FDA to seek the injunction.

Like the audit required under an Applications Integrity Policy, a company may be required by the terms of an injunction to conduct an internal investigation into its procedures, including, for example, procedures for submitting NDAs and NDA supplements and assuring that the data are accurate, authentic, and reliable. Injunction decrees may often require retrospective reviews of procedures and records to reaffirm the validity of data already accepted by the FDA. The decree may also interpose a role for an independent outside consultant to review submissions that have already been endorsed by all appropriate personnel within the company.

In 1995, Eli Lilly & Company entered into a Consent Decree of Permanent Injunction under which it was required to adopt and implement new procedures to ensure that its submission of changes to NDAs complied with FDA regulations, 21 C.F.R. § 314.70. The company was ordered to cease and desist from any practice of nonreporting "simply because, in the unilateral view of Lilly, the change is not, or does not effect, a 'critical parameter' of the drug product in question." The company was required to conduct a comprehensive investigation, through independent consultants, to assess its documentation of production changes and the submission of changes to the FDA. The consent decree also required Lilly to pay $375,000 as reimbursement for the FDA investigation [19].

Such indirect fines are not uncommon. In several recent injunction decrees, companies have agreed to reimburse the government for the cost of the FDA investigation resulting in the discovery of the discrepancies.

Most FDA injunction orders prevent companies from distributing the inventory of the drugs that are subject to the injunction, thus putting those drugs, in effect, under FDA control. The injunction decree will require that the drugs be destroyed or reconditioned under the FDA's supervision and to its satisfaction before they may be released. As an alternative, the FDA can ask the Justice Department to file a separate seizure case against certain drugs.

Another alternative available to the FDA is to refer information for enforcement action by the states. The FDA has developed an active working relationship with the National Association of Attorneys General (NAAG). In fact, the Agency has established an FDA Task Force with the NAAG and procedures for sharing information. Because 46 states have adopted the uniform food and drug law, almost any product deficiency that would support a finding of adulteration or misbranding under the Federal Food, Drug, and Cosmetic Act is also a violation of the state food and drug laws. Moreover, the State Attorneys General have given a high priority to business activities involving fraud. In many cases, several Attorneys General will reach an agreement with a company over practices that the states find objectionable. These agreements often call for the issuance of "Dear Doctor" letters and other corrective measures, training programs for company personnel, fines against the company, and reimbursement for the state's investigative costs. As is apparent, these requirements and sanctions closely parallel those that the FDA seeks to obtain it its federal injunction cases.

For example, in 1993, Sandoz Pharmaceuticals entered a "voluntary compliance agreement" with the Attorneys General of 34 states in which it agreed to stop advertising a brand of its children's cough syrup as "new" or "improved." The company agreed to issue corrective labeling and notifications to both users and retailers. Under the agreement, the company was also required to make refunds to consumers who complained about being misled by the promotional claims. Finally, Sandoz agreed to pay a fine of $800,000.

6. Criminal Investigation and Prosecution

If a pre-approval inspection spills over into a more general FDA investigation that in turn discloses what appears to be knowing or intentional fraudulent conduct or other potential violation of federal criminal laws, the FDA will not hesitate to recommend that the Justice Department pursue its own investigation, with or without the assistance of a federal grand jury, and file criminal charges if warranted [20]. Indeed, for a marketed drug, the range of potential criminal charges is greater because many violations of the Federal Food, Drug, and Cosmetic Act are predicated on a shipment of an adulterated or misbranded drug in interstate commerce, i.e., on the fact that a violative drug is being marketed. Moreover, if marketing of the drug has created a public health risk or serious adverse reaction among users, the likelihood that the Justice Department will pursue criminal charges is greatly increased.

In late 1995, Warner-Lambert plead guilty to failing to notify the FDA about stability problems with one of its approved drugs with the intent to defraud and mislead the Agency [21]. The company was sentenced to pay a fine of $10 million. A Warner-Lambert Quality Assurance official was indicted on charges of causing the interstate shipment of drugs that were adulterated due to the failure of the drugs to meet their stability requirements. The indictment specifically recited:

> FDA's NDA reviewers in Rockville, Maryland, relied on inspectional observations and other information developed by FDA field personnel to determine whether an NDA applicant was operating in conformance with GMP. FDA's NDA reviewers in Rockville, Maryland, also relied on such field-generated information to assess whether grounds existed for undertaking proceedings to withdraw an NDA approval.

The indictment also observed that the Quality Assurance official's responsibilities included notifying the FDA "of any failure of a drug to meet the specifications of its NDA . . . [and] for stopping the shipment of a drug, and initiating a recall (if necessary), when the drug failed to meet the specifications of its NDA. . . ." The quality assurance official was also charged with obstruction for impeding the FDA's administration of the Federal Food, Drug, and Cosmetics Act by concealing from the Agency information concerning the stability test failures and other GMP deficiencies [22].

In announcing the plea and the indictment, the United States Attorney in Baltimore announced that her office "will continue to investigate and prosecute fraud relating to pharmaceutical products, whether by brand name or generic manufacturers."

V. CONCLUSIONS

Most pre-approval inspections go reasonably well. The majority of companies pass the inspection, and the NDA or supplement is approved or at least is not delayed due to adverse inspection findings.

For companies that experience failure, in most cases the consequence will be limited to a delay in approval of the NDA drug accompanied by the need to implement improvements in manufacturing procedures, revalidate data, rerun pilot batches, and/or modify the NDA. By achieving compliance or providing the FDA with reliable data, the company can satisfy the FDA and the product can move forward.

However, in some circumstances, the failure of a pre-approval inspection can begin a cascade of events, resulting in administrative, civil, and criminal sanctions. The imposition of these sanctions can and usually does have a significant adverse impact on the company and its employees. Moreover, the events supporting the imposition of these sanctions can seriously diminish the credibility of the company in the eyes of the FDA. Indeed, in the last analysis, losing the confidence of the FDA may be the most significant and pervasive adverse consequence of failing a pre-approval inspection.

NOTES

1. According to the FDA's *Compliance Program Guide For Pre-Approval Inspections (Compliance Program 7346.382)*, the role of the FDA District Office in pre-approval inspections is to: (1) assess GMP compliance, (2) verify the authenticity and accuracy of the data supporting the application, and (3) to assess any other data that may impact on a firm's ability to manufacture a drug in compliance with GMPs. District investigators are also instructed to determine whether differences between representations in the NDA and documents and procedures at the company may constitute fraud, to assess whether the application misrepresents data, and to explore other inconsistencies and/or deficiencies that raise significant questions about the validity of records. District Offices are instructed that they should recommend withholding approval when significant deviations from GMPs are observed or when there are other significant failures to meet the application commitments.
2. 21 C.F. R. § 312.53(a).
3. 56 Fed. Reg. 46,191.
4. Under the *Points to Consider*, the audit plan should have seven elements: (1) an analysis of the audit findings, including identification of all individuals who were or may have been associated with or involved in the wrongful acts and identification of defective practices, procedures, products, and applications; (2) the disposition of any recommendations by the audit consultant; (3) a description of the actions taken and to be taken to achieve correction; (4) a timetable for implementing corrective actions; (5) identification of the persons responsible for assuring the satisfactory and timely implementation of the corrective action plan; (6) the creation of a comprehensive ethics program to prevent recurrence of similar wrongdoing; and (7) procedures for monitoring the effectiveness of the plan.
5. 21 U.S.C. § 335a(a)(2).
6. 21 U.S.C. § 335a(k).
7. 21 U.S.C. § 335b.
8. 21 U.S.C. § 335a(b). In addition, an individual may be debarred if he or she has been convicted of a federal misdemeanor or a state law felony for conduct relating to the

development or approval of any drug subject to FDA approval or relating to "the regulation of" any such drug, and the FDA concludes that the conduct undermined the process of the regulation for drugs. An individual may also be debarred if convicted of a felony involving fraud, false statements, falsification or destruction of records, or interference with or obstruction of an investigation into such matters, or if he or she has been convicted of conspiracy to engage in any of these felonies if the FDA also finds that the individual has demonstrated "a pattern of conduct sufficient to find that there is reason to believe that such individual may violate" requirements imposed under the Federal Food, Drug, and Cosmetic Act relating to drugs.

9. 21 U.S.C. § 335a(b)(2)(B).
10. 21 U.S.C. § 335a(i).
11. 21 U.S.C. § 335a(e).
12. The FDA published a "functional statement" for the Office in the *Federal Register* on December 27, 1991. *See* 56 Fed. Reg. 67,076.
13. *See*, 21 C.F.R. Part 20.108 as amended by publication in the *Federal Register* on September 20, 1993.
14. 21 U.S.C. § 374(a).
15. *See*, *Department of Justice Health Care Fraud Report*, Fiscal Year 1994.
16. *See*, 21 C.F.R. Part 7.
17. *See*, 21 U.S.C. § 334.
18. *See*, 21 U.S.C. § 332.
19. The decree declares that no criminal prosecution will be brought against Lilly for any failure to comply with the reporting and premarket approval requirements, except, however, if a fraudulent intent or willful misconduct were to be discovered.
20. The same investigative techniques, evidence development procedures, and FDA/ Department of Justice coordination as described in Section III of this chapter apply.
21. 21 U.S.C. §§ 331(e); 333(a)(2).
22. *See*, 18 U.S.C. § 1505.
23. These criminal proceedings in 1995 were preceded by Warner-Lambert entering into a Consent Decree of Permanent Injunction in 1993, focusing on compliance with GMPs and adherence to FDA requirements for NDA drugs.

6

Successful Management of a Pre-Approval Inspection

Paul E. Wray
International Pharmaceutical Services, Bridgewater, New Jersey

I. INTRODUCTION

This chapter discusses management of the Food and Drug Administration (FDA) audit, which is called the new drug application (NDA) pre-approval inspection (PAI). Between January/February 1990 and February 1992, I was involved with 16 PAIs as an executive in a major pharmaceutical company. In this capacity, either I or another designated person participated in the PAI to provide the scale-up and validation expertise for the particular NDA under review. Between March 1992 and February 1996, I participated directly or indirectly in another 20 PAIs as a consultant to the NDA sponsor firm. In four of these PAIs, I was in direct contact with the FDA auditor. In the remainder of the PAIs, my role was to help prepare the firm for all aspects of the PAI and to advise the sponsor during the PAI "from behind the scenes." For each of the above PAIs I was also involved with any Report of Adverse Findings (form 483) that resulted from the audit. Of the more than 35 PAIs, although most resulted in the receipt of a form 483, none were judged nonapprovable, and therefore did not impact the review and approval of the NDA under consideration.

"Management" of an NDA PAI implies that one exerts control over the inspection and has the ability to influence the outcome of the inspection. It is indeed possible to have that effect on the PAI, and this chapter discusses how to do it.

It is not possible to tell the FDA auditor what to do, what to request to see, what documents to examine, what copies to take, and what issues to examine in depth. The management that we can introduce into the PAI is anticipating the FDA requirements, minimizing unexpected FDA issues, and developing strategies for selected issues in advance, thereby influencing or "managing" the PAI and minimizing the potential for a PAI to become "out of control."

The following aspects of the PAI are discussed in this chapter. The first aspect is the timing of the PAI. It is useful to establish a window of time during which the PAI will most probably occur so that you can plan for the audit. Factors that can influence the date of the audit and assist in forecasting the most probable window of time for the audit are presented.

This chapter also describes the most likely format of a PAI audit, including the normal sequence of events that the FDA tends to follow. Knowing what to expect enables better planning. This also results in confidence—an important trait. In addition to the format of the audit, this chapter discusses the advance preparation needed to manage the auditor. How should the FDA auditor be received at the company? Where should the auditor be located during the audit? Who should meet with the auditor during the audit? What records need to be kept during the audit? What type of support personnel is required during the audit? How do you organize the records that you expect the FDA to request during the audit? What type of training should be considered before the audit? Each of these issues can be a potential problem in an audit.

A discussion of the raw data review is also included. One of the primary assignments of the FDA during the PAI is to authenticate the data that have been included in the NDA. There are several predictable types of data that the FDA auditor will review. These data are discussed here, and the advance preparation of these data for the audit is reviewed in depth. The raw data review aspect of the PAI has consistently been one of the most problematic issues for firms experiencing a PAI; therefore, specific advice on how to improve your firm's state of preparedness is outlined. Special attention is also given to drug substance and drug product stability data. These data are almost always reviewed during the PAI, and they will also be reviewed by the chemist who is handling the NDA review at the FDA Drug Division in Rockville, MD. This "double review" puts extra pressure on these data; therefore, there is extra discussion on how to successfully withstand the division review as well as the audit. The internal auditing of the above data is also discussed, along with specific recommendations with regard to practicing raw data retrieval and training of personnel to perform raw data retrieval.

A discussion of development history is also included. Currently, NDAs are required to contain information that justifies the formula and process for the commercial product. This information is usually included in the CM&C section of the NDA and is relatively brief. However, for the PAI it can be anticipated that the

FDA auditor will expect the firm to have detailed information available to track the product development from clinical phase I through clinical phase III and on to the commercial formula and process.

Recommendations are made regarding the best way to satisfy this expectation and how this information can lead logically to and be very supportive of the product process validation. Process validation is covered in other chapters in this book; however, options for when the firm should manufacture these three validation batches are discussed here. Obviously, they must be completed before commercialization, after the NDA is approved. However, there are options as to how early these batches are manufactured. Regardless of when your firm chooses to make the requisite validation batches, you must have the Process Validation Protocol available and approved before the trials, and ready to show to the FDA auditor during the PAI. Therefore, this chapter includes a discussion of the process validation protocol.

The penultimate section of this chapter reviews the FDA expectations regarding technology transfer. It is very clear that the FDA has consistent concerns that the NDA sponsor has manufactured the commercial formula using the process, equipment, and site specified in the NDA. In addition, they will assess that the production personnel have been adequately trained to assume the responsibility for the manufacture of the commercial batches after the NDA is approved. The lack of transferring the technology to the production unit and documenting that occurrence has been cited by the FDA in form 483s. This chapter discusses how to perform the technology transfer and how to document it so as to satisfy this requirement. All firms should conduct technology transfer even if the FDA were not concerned. The optimum sequence of events including technology transfer and process validation and the coordination of these activities is described.

This chapter ends with the discussion of the FDA form 483. This Notice of Adverse Findings is, more often than not, the final report that the firm will receive at the completion of the PAI. This chapter discusses the appropriate attitude for a firm to take when it receives a 483, and how to prepare in advance to move rapidly through this exchange with the FDA. This also can be managed if the firm develops strategies and prepares responses in advance of the receipt of a 483. This chapter ends with a discussion of when a firm should agree with the FDA and make the requested changes or improvements, and when a stand should be taken that is in opposition to the FDA district auditor.

II. TIMING OF THE PAI

The PAI clock will start running when your NDA has been filed with the FDA. However, your filing date is not the day you send the NDA to the FDA. When the

FDA receives a new submission, it performs an evaluation for "completeness." This preliminary evaluation does not constitute a review, but is merely a determination of whether all the NDA content requirements have been met. The NDA will be sent to each of the FDA reviewing disciplines, such as chemist, pharmacologist, etc., who will ultimately review the submission, and they will take 30 to 45 days to assess the completeness of the particular portion of the NDA that they will be responsible for during the full review. After approximately 45 days, a meeting will be held within the FDA, and each reviewer will report the results of their findings. If the submission is complete, the FDA will accept it and the formal review will begin. The NDA firm will be formally notified by the FDA via a letter that their NDA has been accepted for review. The acceptance of the NDA by the FDA starts the clock for the PAI. However, if the submission is judged to be deficient, the FDA will notify the firm of its options. The FDA will not review the NDA if it is judged incomplete or deficient, and the PAI clock will not begin. This is known as Refusal to File (RTF).

After the PAI clock begins, it is expected that the FDA District Office will contact the sponsor firm within approximately 45 days to notify the firm of the pending PAI. The District Office will ascertain that the firm is ready for the PAI, and if the firm responds favorably, the schedule for the PAI could be mutually set. However, usually the FDA District Office will not set a date at this time. It is customary that, once it has been established that the firm is ready, the PAI not be announced in advance and the district inspector or inspectors will arrive to start the inspection when they desire, based on their schedule. The firm could respond to the FDA that they are not ready; however, not having the capability to manufacture the NDA drug product is not an acceptable reason. Acceptable reasons include the following: (1) completion of process validation; or (2) completion of cleaning validation. A firm should not tell the FDA that they are not ready, but if a delay in the PAI would permit the firm to complete the above activities, it would make the FDA's job easier to wait and conduct the inspection when the validations are complete, rather than being in the position of having to return at a later date to review the validation reports.

The earliest probable date for the PAI is, based on the previously mentioned considerations, approximately 45 days after the NDA is accepted for filing by the FDA. The absolute latest date for the PAI is just before the final NDA approval. If the NDA review and approval takes the typical 24 months, then the PAI could occur within a "window" that is approximately 24 months long. This is typically not the case, but it does happen. Recently, the FDA has conducted the PAI within 6 months of the start of the NDA review, and few go beyond 12 months after the filing date. Therefore, for planning purposes, a PAI window of 12 months after the NDA filing is recommended, with the highest probability for the PAI being within 6 months after filing.

There are a number of factors that can cause deviation from this planning schedule. If your firm and the primary manufacturing facility in the NDA have never been inspected, the FDA tends to inspect earlier rather than later. If your firm and the primary manufacturing facility in the NDA are due for the biannual current Good Manufacturing Practices (cGMP) inspection, then the FDA will tend to perform both the PAI and biannual cGMP inspection during the same visit. The FDA will therefore need to set aside more time for the inspection, which could delay the events. If your firm has had the primary manufacturing facility inspected recently, the FDA could delay the PAI, especially if the previous inspection was favorable. If your firm has established a very good track record in previous PAIs, e.g., six consecutive successful PAIs, the FDA has stated that they could consider not inspecting for this NDA. Other things also influence the scheduling of the PAI, including the time of year (holidays or vacations), whether the FDA was "in the area," a field complaint, or the review chemist having a particular issue they want the field to examine.

If the NDA has multiple manufacturing and packaging sites, the FDA will usually inspect the primary site first and then the others in order of importance, based on their potential impact on product quality. If the NDA has X-U.S. sites for manufacture of either drug substance or drug product, those inspections are performed by the International Division and in addition to the above considerations are impacted by the FDA travel budgets and travel time. As a generalization, the X-U.S. sites take longer to be inspected than the U.S. sites.

III. THE PAI AUDIT FORMAT

The audit format includes two aspects: (1) where the audit will probably occur; and (2) what will be audited. Before discussing these two aspects, it is important to consider managing the format of the PAI. This is performed by planning all aspects of the audit, including greeting the auditor (who and how), logistics of the location of the room for the FDA auditor, firm representatives to interface with the auditor and their roles, staff to support the individuals in the room with the auditor, copy facility, etc. The person who greets the FDA auditor should remain with the auditor for the duration of the audit. It is also important to designate a back-up individual in case of illness or emergency. A private room close to the entrance and to restrooms should be chosen for the audit. The room does not need a phone and should not be on the public announcement system. The room should not have views of the facility or hallway. It can have windows to the outside. Ideally, there should be an adjacent room for the personnel who are supporting the firm representatives in the room with the auditor. The room should have plenty of working space for up to four people and should be comfortable with good HVAC.

Routes from the audit room to all potential sites of inspection within the facility should be planned.

Regarding where the audit will probably occur, the firm must expect that each manufacturing site specified in the NDA will be audited, including (1) the bulk drug substance site; (2) the drug product; and (3) the packaging site. If there are multiple sites for any or all of the above, the firm must plan for each of them to be audited. The FDA will also audit whether the site is in the U.S. or X-U.S. The format for the PAI consists of a number of absolutes, items that the FDA always reviews, and a larger number of highly probable items. In addition, there are items for which a firm should always be prepared, even though they are seldom audited.

The PAI will almost always include an in-depth review of the batch records for pivotal clinical and stability batches. Some of these batch records may be included in the NDA, and the others will be in the firm's files. The FDA will review these records because they represent the "decision makers" in the NDA. These batch records will be reviewed from several aspects. They will first be reviewed for their GMP quality. Are the batch records correctly completed? Are the batch records completely supported by all other documentation (i.e., weigh tickets, equipment logs, personnel training records, etc.)? Are all of the calculations in the batch records correct? Is raw data available to support the batch records? Next, they will be reviewed side by side with the NDA to ascertain whether the formula and process is the same as that filed in the NDA. If the comparison shows that the pivotal batches are identical to the NDA with regard to formula and process, the auditor will go on to other issues. However, if the batch records for the pivotal batches reveal differences, the auditor will stay with this issue until he or she is convinced that there has been adequate work performed to show comparability.

The differences between the NDA and the pivotal batches can be found in one of the three different regards. First, the formulas are different. The most common example of this is when the company uses hard gelatin capsules for clinical material up to late phase III, and then switches to the desired commercial form, e.g., a tablet. The firm must have data to support the comparability between the NDA product and the clinical product. The data must include: (1) chemical stability; (2) physical stability; (3) dissolution; and possibly (4) clinical efficacy or bioavailability. If the differences between the NDA and clinical batches are not significant, the amount of data can be minimal. The firm must use its best objective judgment in this regard.

Second, the process could differ between the NDA and the clinical batches. This is a very typical disparity and is usually the result of product process scale-up and optimization. The data to document comparability is very similar to that needed for the above case: (1) chemical stability; (2) physical stability; and (3) dissolution.

If the dosage form is of the immediate release (IR) type, the firm should consult the SUPAC guidelines for assistance in determining the significance of the process change. For other types of dosage forms, the best advice is to try to get an early read on the possible FDA concerns for this difference by including this issue in the "end of phase II" meeting with the FDA before filing the NDA.

Lastly, both the formula and process of the clinical batches may differ from those specified in the NDA. This is often the case for a firm performing clinical trials on hard gelatin capsule material and switching to the commercial form late in phase III, as discussed in the first case. However, because the formula and process have both been changed, the proof of comparability is more difficult, and will require: (1) chemical stability; (2) physical stability; (3) dissolution; and very probably (4) clinical efficacy. These issues should be discussed with the FDA at the pre-NDA meeting, before filing the NDA. This will enable the firm to plan and conduct the necessary trials to document the issue of comparability, and the possibility of the FDA reviewing chemist or PAI auditor raising these issues will be avoided.

In addition to the pivotal batch records, the PAI format will usually include a review of the raw data for the above batches. The subject of raw data review is very important and is discussed in depth later in this chapter. However, for purposes of discussing audit format, it must be briefly included now. Specifically, the auditor would be expected to examine the data associated with the release testing of these batches. This would also include the data for the release of the drug substance, the excipients for these batches, and the stability data on these batches. This data trail could also lead to the analytical method validation reports for each of the analytical methods involved. Additionally, if the release testing for the drug product required dissolution testing, the dissolution raw data as well as the method validation reports for the analytical method used in dissolution testing could be reviewed.

To expedite and manage the audit of the above batch records and raw data, it is recommended that copies of all of these documents and data be assembled at one site, preferably the primary manufacturing site. However, if multiple sites are specified in the NDA, plans must be made for the transfer of all of this information to each of the PAI sites. It is in the firm's best interest, and greatly facilitates the PAI, to provide any requested information promptly. The above information will probably be requested, and the ready availability on site will expedite the inspection and create a very positive impression on the auditor.

The review of the batch records and the associated data leads the auditor to the next two probable items of the PAI. The discussion of the evolution of the formula and process, as depicted by the differences observed between the early developmental batches used in clinical material, and the final formula and process documented in the NDA, can best be explained and defended by use of a development history. This document is very important for the PAI, and its format and content is discussed in depth later in this chapter. It is mentioned here because this would be the natural place for it to be used in the audit.

The other probable issue at this time would be the facility specified in the NDA. The typical format of a PAI will include a GMP inspection of the facility and equipment used to manufacture this product as specified in the NDA. This inspection will require the auditor to leave the conference room being used for the PAI and go to the production site. To effectively manage this portion of the PAI, the firm must have readied the production site for this inspection. This is of primary importance, but it is also wise to plan in advance for the walk to the production area. The auditor should be taken by the most advantageous route. It is very clear that the auditor can and will see everything they wish, but plan the route of this walk to the firm's advantage. Put your best foot forward. Clean, paint, and ready this area in addition to the production area.

The PAI inspection of the manufacturing site is best described as a typical GMP inspection. It will be product-specific and will focus on the equipment and facility used for the NDA product. However, if the auditor is also going to conduct a biannual cGMP inspection, as discussed earlier, it would happen at this time. Emphasis would be placed on the new NDA product, but would also cover all the typical aspects of the biannual inspection. On the other hand, if the inspector is performing only a PAI, which is product-specific, he or she can and will change it to a full cGMP inspection if there are issues revealed during the PAI that raise concern. For this to happen, the auditor would need to find issues that are globally problematic such as standard operating procedures (SOPs) or general house-keeping. There can be product-specific issues that do not have broader implica-tions, and these could be addressed in the PAI; however, if there are systemic concerns about the equipment and facility used for the NDA product, the auditor could decide to perform an in-depth cGMP inspection on the spot.

To manage this unexpected event, the firm should perform internal audits annually, as well as a mock PAI for this product before the actual event. These audits, if performed well, should prevent unexpected inspection findings. Internal auditing could be difficult for a small firm with limited staff. The importance of these audits justifies the use of outside assistance from special consultants. It is not advised that an organization audit itself. The auditor must be independent or, at the very least, from another group in the company. Internal, nonindependent results are suspect. It is also vital that the internal or consultant audits be acted upon and the deficiencies corrected before the PAI.

Another highly probable audit issue is process validation and cleaning valida-tion. There are three circumstances that need to be discussed in this regard: (1) the firm could have completed the process and cleaning validation trials before the NDA submission; (2) the firm could plan to perform the validation trials after the

NDA is submitted but before the PAI; and (3) the firm could plan to perform the trials after the PAI but before NDA approval. Each of these options is followed by various firms. Few firms have the time or money to complete the validation before the NDA submission, and there is a very high probability that the drug product made during these trials will expire before NDA approval. This does have the clear advantage of minimizing any doubt with regard to the validatibility of the NDA formula and process. It also will enable the auditor to review these trials during the PAI and eliminate the need of a return visit, for review of this work, before the NDA approval. It should be noted that for sterile products, the FDA now wants the process validation to be completed and included in the NDA. If a firm's NDA is being "fast tracked," this option would be best. For other dosage forms, there are the two other options.

The second option has several advantages and disadvantages. The advantages include: having the work completed for the review by the PAI auditor, thereby precluding a second FDA visit; not having to expend the time and money during the hectic NDA preparation time; and having a higher probability of the drug product manufactured for the validation trials not expiring, and being saleable material. The primary disadvantage is the compressed timing within which the trials must be performed. It would be expected that these trials would require 3 to 5 months to complete. If the PAI happens before 3 months, which is possible, the work would not be completed and the firm would now be under option three and have the downside of not having validation complete at the time of the PAI.

The third option, performing the validation trials after the PAI but before the expected NDA approval date, is the most popular choice by pharmaceutical firms. The main reason for choosing this option seems to be financial. The value of three or more full-scale batches, and their potential loss due to expiry dating, does not offset the downside of a potential second audit visit before NDA approval.

The option selected by the firm will determine the audit format at this stage of the PAI. If the firm has all of the validation work completed, the FDA auditor will review the reports and audit the raw data. The batch records for these trials will also be audited for GMP concerns, as well as compared with the NDA formula and process. These trials must conform closely to the NDA, with any disparities supported by appropriate documentation.

If the firm has not performed the validation trials, it should have approved process and cleaning validation protocols available for the auditor to review. Allowing the FDA auditor to review these documents at this time will give the firm time to make any revisions or adjustments that the auditor could request. The revised protocols would then be used to conduct these trials, and the firm would have high confidence that the validation trials would be found acceptable as a result of the prior FDA protocol review. This FDA review may also allow the auditor the possibility of reviewing the validation reports at their office rather than coming to the firm, since they previously reviewed the protocols. The Process Validation protocol and the Cleaning Validation Protocol are two important documents for the PAI. They are discussed in depth later in this chapter. It will be shown that they are the link between the development history and the NDA formula and process.

The PAI audit format will be affected by the training and experience of the auditors. The FDA attempts to match the training and experiences of the auditors to the firm and NDA. The FDA PAI team will probably consist of at least two auditors. One of the two auditors will probably be experienced in cGMP inspections, and the other would probably be a scientist. It would be expected that the two inspectors would often work separately. The cGMP inspector could be performing the facility and equipment audit, while the other inspector could be reviewing reports and raw data. If the auditors work separately, the firm must be prepared to have a representative with each auditory constantly.

After the above aspects have been addressed, the audit format will be determined by issues that have concerned the auditor. It is often possible to predict what the auditor is concerned with and have some time to prepare for an in-depth review of a particular aspect. This is done by (1) noting when the auditors write; (2) what questions the auditors ask; (3) what copies the auditors take; and (4) what the auditors may be willing to share with the firm at the end of each day. The firm must ask for this feedback. Some auditors will be more open than others, and the general attitude of the inspectors is to help the firm improve. Therefore, they may want to discuss concerns with the firm so that changes can be initiated as soon as possible.

In discussing the audit format, it is important to note that the sequence of items is very hard to predict. What has been discussed is what will be reviewed, but not necessarily in the order that items will be reviewed.

IV. THE RAW DATA REVIEW

The primary reason that the FDA NDA PAI program was initiated was because of fraudulent data. Therefore, one of the specific assignments that the auditors bring to the firm is to authenticate the data in the NDA. The authentification is accomplished by finding the raw data and confirming that it is legitimate. This section discusses what data will be reviewed, the strategy of preparing for the raw data review, what comprises the raw data trail, and what type of inspection will be performed on the laboratories that generated the analytical data.

The primary source of raw data in the NDA is the chemical stability of the various lots of drug product and the lots of drug substance that are presented in the NDA. These data are included in support of the requested expiry dating of the drug product. It is also included to document the drug product composition and quality that was used in the various clinical studies in the submission. In addition to the chemical stability data, data obtained from the release testing of each of the clinical batches and for each lot of the drug substance that was used in the clinical and stability batches are popular targets. If the firm has performed process and cleaning validation, those data would also probably be audited.

After the raw data review for the above data, it is probable that the raw data contained in all of the analytical method validation reports would be authenticated. These data support the precision, accuracy, linearity, sensitivity, etc., of the analytical methods. If problems are revealed in these validation data, the stability, batch release, and validation data would come into question.

Another probable raw data source that would be audited is the batch records for all of the batches contained in the NDA, including chemical assay results, physical test results, weighing determinations, and calculations.

Considering the probable data targets, how should the firm prepare for the raw data audit? The problem all firms face is that of the age of the raw data records. Many years elapse during the preparation of an NDA. People are hired, other people leave, methods change, technology changes, and all of these events must be documented and filed so as to be retrieved. All of the data, from all the sources delineated above, should be collected and audited internally before the submission of the NDA.

After the data have been audited and corrections have been noted, the firm must designate a person to be responsible for raw data retrieval for the FDA auditor. This individual or individuals must then practice raw data retrieval under simulated conditions. The firm representative must not only be able to find the raw data, but must be able to explain how to interpret the data, if necessary. The firm should not call upon individual chemists to explain their laboratory notebooks. Instead, individual chemists should train the selected representatives to explain the notebooks or reports. If the analytical chemist has left the firm, the representative must have time to interpret these notebooks in advance of the PAI. With proper advance preparation and practice, it is possible to avoid problems with the raw data trail. Because of the importance of this issue, the firm should train a back-up to the primary representative. The proficiency of the firm in retrieving raw data and explaining it to the FDA auditor is the basis of much of the FDA impression of the firm. A good job creates a good impression, and the reverse is also true.

V. THE DEVELOPMENT HISTORY

Drafting a formal development history for a new drug product became necessary in the early 1990s. In approximately 1991, the FDA started requesting that the development history be included in the CM&C section of the NDA to facilitate the audit. This requirement has never been clarified or codified to any extent by the agency. The industry has tried to satisfy the various FDA requirements and desires with documents that are (1) not consistent from company to company and (2) not consistent from drug product to drug product for a given company.

The purpose that this report fulfills in the NDA is to help the FDA review chemist to understand the science and technology that went into the development of this new product. European regulatory authorities have required a Development Pharmaceutics report for several years. The FDA was aware of this and realized that such a document, if well written, would enable the review chemist to better understand the drug product and make more intelligent judgements about this product during the review process. The recommended basic content of this document for inclusion in the NDA is as follows: (1) justify the purpose of each of the ingredients in the formula; (2) justify the amounts of each ingredient in the formula; (3) describe the evolution of the manufacturing process; (4) justify the final process in the NDA; and (5) document which of the manufacturing process steps are deemed "critical" and which are not, so as to support the process validation that must be performed before commercialization.

Considering the content of the document, it becomes apparent that this is a very demanding and time-consuming requirement. The most difficult aspect is assembling the development information, which can span several years. When the development history was first introduced into the NDA, companies tended to write very long and complicated documents. The feedback that the FDA is giving now is that the document should be brief and reader-friendly. To achieve this, the use of spread sheets is recommended, with concise verbiage to lead the reviewer through the document. Examples of these spread sheets are discussed in this chapter. An outline of the content of a typical development history report is given in Table 1.

The drug substance preformulation studies should begin with an adequate characterization of the drug substance. This characterization data would lead to the elimination of some excipients because of obvious incompatibilities. The remaining excipients under consideration would be subjected to screening studies, leading to selection of final choices. The quantities of the ingredients should also be addressed. This information will justify the formula of the drug product.

The process is justified by presenting the history of the process development that leads to the selection of the final process. The report would then document the final formula and process that is filed in the NDA. Next, the scale-up history and the identification of the critical process steps, and why they are critical steps, would be described. The establishment of acceptance criteria for the critical steps will come from the data developed during the scale-up experience.

Table 1 Outline of a Typical Development History Report

Topic	Reason
Preformulation of drug substance	Screening of excipients
Selection of excipients	Formula justification
Process development history	Process justification
Selection of final formula and process	Support for NDA
Scale-up to production scale	Support for NDA
Critical process steps	Support for validation
Acceptance criteria—critical steps	Support for validation
Discussion of pivotal batches	Assist FDA review chemist

The development history report would close with a concise discussion of the pivotal batches that were the "decision makers" during the formula and process finalization. This discussion will help the FDA review chemist to understand the drug product. It should be noted that this report has now put all the support in place for the Process Validation Protocol, which is a very important document to have available for the PAI. The format and content of this document is discussed in another chapter. However, to have your firm in the best possible position for the pending PAI, it is strongly recommended that the Process Validation Protocol be written and approved before the audit. During the PAI, at the optimal time, the protocol should be discussed with the auditors. The purpose of the discussion is to ascertain any problems or deficiencies in the protocol that the auditors would discuss with the firm, and then to revise the protocol, if necessary, before performing the validation trials.

This process has two major benefits. The first benefit is that the FDA auditor could make helpful recommendations concerning the protocol and add to its acceptability. The validation trials that will subsequently be performed under this improved protocol will have an increased chance of being found acceptable. The second benefit is that it may reduce the need of the FDA auditor to return to the firm to audit the validation results just before shipping product to trade (commercialization) of the new approved NDA. If the auditors have had a chance to review the protocol (during the PAI), and agree with what the firm proposes in the protocol, they may feel comfortable reviewing the process validation reports in the FDA offices rather than returning to the firm a second time. This would be a significant gain and help in the management of the audit.

The development history report also has an important purpose in the PAI. If properly written, this document will help the firm to explain the new product to the PAI auditor. The PAI auditor at the firm needs to fully understand the product and its formula and process to facilitate the PAI and subsequent recommendations from the auditor with regard to the firm's approvability or nonapprovability. It is also recommended that the firm plan a brief formal presentation to the PAI auditors at the beginning of the PAI. The development history report is an ideal document to use during this presentation. It will give the auditors a concise review of the NDA product and give each reviewer (assuming there are more than one) the same information at the same time so that they all start with the same understanding.

The development history can be viewed as having two distinct formats. The one for the CM&C section of the NDA would be brief and inclusive of only critical trials, while the format of the document available at the firm for use during the PAI would be complete and very comprehensive. One could view the NDA development history as a summary of the development history available at the firm. Both review chemists and PAI auditors have expressed the same need for the information contained in the development history, but the review chemist often values brevity, while the auditor needs to see all of the development activities. These disparate needs can be met if the document included in the NDA is a summary of the document made available to the auditor during the PAI. Obviously, the two documents must be consistent with each other, but this can be accomplished as well as satisfying the two FDA divisions if the above recommendations are considered.

VI. THE TECHNOLOGY TRANSFER

Scale-up from laboratory scale to pilot scale and on to production scale should occur during the development phase of the new product. The NDA should contain data from pivotal trials that were manufactured at pilot and production scale. If an NDA does not contain data from production scale trials, it is not complete. Therefore, the development history report should include not less than one (three are optimum) production scale trials. The data from these trials provide the basis for the Process Validation Protocol.

After these tasks are complete, the next step is Process Validation and Technology Transfer. These are listed together because it is recommended that they be accomplished at the same time. Both are requirements of FDA that must be satisfied before final NDA approval and commercialization (interstate shipment). Process Validation is covered in detail in another chapter of this book. Technology Transfer is the last step in the transfer of the product from Research and Development to Production. Technology Transfer has three basic elements. First, a document that represents the Production manufacturing record is prepared. It is called many things by various companies, but here it is referred to as the

Master Batch Record (MBR). This MBR should be identical in content to the CM&C section of the NDA. Many firms include a copy of this document in the NDA as a representative batch record. This document is used during the technology transfer event.

The second basic element of technology transfer is the actual manufacture of the production batches. These batches would be manufactured at full scale using the NDA formula and process in the commercial manufacturing facility with the equipment train that is specified in the NDA. The batches should be manufactured under the supervision of both Research and Development and Production and performed by production operators as a training opportunity.

The FDA requires that these events be documented completely so as to demonstrate that the product is manufacturable by the firm in the commercial facility using the production operators. The following sequence of events is recommended to accomplish both the process validation and technology transfer: (1) Research and Development writes the Process Validation Protocol and has it approved by management personnel from Research and Development and Production. (2) The validation batches are set up and performed (three consecutive, successful trials) using the MBR and above protocol. (3) Production operators are trained during the three trials, and their training is documented. (4) The Process Validation Report is written, and it is approved by the same three management personnel (Research and Development, Quality Control/Quality Assurance, and Production).

After the completion of these trials, a brief Technology Transfer report should be written, using the above documents as appendixes. This report documents that Production approved and participated in the validation trials and also completed technology transfer at the same time, and eliminates the need for a separate technology transfer event and more batches. All FDA requirements are met if documentation of the above-described series of events is completed. It should be noted that Cleaning Validation could also be performed between these three trials with proper planning and coordination between production and Research and Development. This is strongly recommended because it saves time and money.

VII. RESPONDING TO FDA 483 ISSUES

Most of the time, the firm will receive a Summary of Adverse Findings, or FDA form 483, at the end of the PAI. In addition, more than one sixth (greater than 17%) of the firms will find themselves nonapprovable and have the NDA review and approval delayed until the issues cited in the 483 are resolved to the satisfaction of the FDA (1).

After PAI has proceeded and the FDA auditors have ended the inspection phase, the auditor will schedule the exit interview. The FDA inspectors usually require 2 to 3 days to prepare for the exit interview. It will be scheduled with the firm on the last day of the actual inspection.

It is recommended that the firm use the 2- to 3-day interval between the end of the audit and the exit interview for strategizing and planning. It is not recommended that you wait until the actual event.

All individuals who participated with the FDA audit should meet to discuss all of the known issues. Once all of the issues are on the table, they should be prioritized in terms of their potential impact on the approvability of the firm. The highest priority is given to the issues that are of highest potential negative impact on approvability. Strategies are established for each of the high-priority issues and probable responses are discussed. This will enable the firm to collect data, reports, etc., that may be not readily available. This is important because it will enable the firm to be more confident at the exit interview and also to respond more rapidly to the 483. The FDA requires that the firm respond within 10 days to the 483, but it is recommended that the firm respond as rapidly as possible; advance preparation will make that possible.

It is very important that the firm does not become adversarial when it receives a 483 during the PAI. Regardless of the circumstances, whether the 483 was totally unjustified or not, the outward appearance of all individuals involved with the FDA during the receipt of the 483 must appear unaffected and not angry. The FDA auditors will complete the inspection and set a date for their return for the exit interview. The firm should assemble a group composed of all those who interacted with the auditor during the inspection and who have been participating in the preparation for the exit interview. The room should be large enough to comfortably seat all participants. The FDA auditors should be introduced to everyone present.

The FDA inspectors will give the appropriate individual at the firm a copy of the 483. Copies of the 483 should be made for all attendees. Next, the FDA will present the issues cited in the 483. During the presentation, it is recommended that only the firm representative who hosted the inspection ask questions for clarification to make sure that there are no misunderstandings. Others should not talk to the auditor during this event.

Disagreements can be expressed, but only in a nonadversarial manner. The auditor will often cite the firm for an issue that was discussed completely during the audit. The firm may have thought that the issue was over, but the auditor has included it in the 483 for completeness. It is appropriate that the item be discussed during the exit interview and that the auditor be reminded about previous documentation and agreements that were reached. However, it will still be necessary for the firm to formally respond to the 483 citation and repeat everything that was previously communicated to the auditor during the inspection.

Overall, the best attitude to maintain during the exit interview is one of "let's work this out together" (firm and FDA). The dominant attitude of the FDA auditor is one of helpfulness and not that of policeman. During any inspection, there will be times when the firm or the FDA will be inclined to take a position that disturbs the other party. These are the times when the firm's advance planning and strategizing will be of greatest benefit. The firm will have decided ahead of time at the strategy meetings where they can "yield" and where they must "stand." This advance planning will be obvious to the FDA auditors, and they generally respond favorably to a firm that is well prepared and has thought through their liabilities and strengths. The firm will yield on issues that reflect their weaknesses, but stand firm on issues that are strengths. This is a reflection of the firm "managing the PAI."

An example of the above is as follows: the firm listed two packaging sites in the NDA, only one of which actually has the capability to perform the required packaging. The auditor cites the firm for not validating the packaging sites and also for the second site not being "capable." The firm's response, which was established ahead of time, would be that they will validate the primary packaging site as requested and withdraw the second site at this time. A response of this type would reflect both flexibility and strength on the firm's part, which would result in a positive relationship with the auditor.

Responses to the 483 issues should be given verbally in the exit interview, unless there are unexpected issues. The verbal responses will then be formalized in the 483 written responses as soon as possible after the exit interview. If there are unexpected issues presented by the FDA auditor during the 483 exit interview, the firm should respond to the auditor immediately, typically with "we will consider your citation and get back to you as soon as possible." These unexpected issues are also the ones that necessitate questioning the auditor until clear understandings are achieved.

Before the end of the exit interview, both the firm and the auditor should know exactly what to expect from each other. The auditor should know what the responses, at least verbally, to the 483 issues are so they are able to assess their adequacy. On the other hand, and more importantly, the firm will know fairly clearly whether they are approvable based on the auditors comments to the verbal responses that the firm has made to the 483 issues. This point in the PAI is a very crucial one. Every effort, within reason, must be made by the firm to help the auditor reach the decision that the firm is approvable for this PAI. The exit interview should not end with the firm having uncertainty over this vital issue. If the firm concludes that the auditor finds them nonapprovable, they must determine the issues creating this conclusion and address them at this time.

If there is latitude on the part of the firm over a particular issue, it should be yielded at this time. If the issue is insurmountable within the 10-day period, both parties should be aware of this. If the issue needs to be appealed to the auditors' supervisor for resolution, the firm should advise the auditor at this time. The firm should tell the auditor exactly what to expect from them in the written responses, and conversely, the firm needs to obtain totally clear issues in the 483 from the auditor.

However, it must be repeated, that in all of the above exchanges, the firm's spokesperson should not become adversarial or argumentative. Additionally, other firm representatives may ask questions for clarification, but only the official firm representative should discuss contentious issues and express agreements and disagreements. The firm should not "gang-up" on the auditor.

The last issue of this chapter is the toughest one: when to give in and when not to give in. This question cannot be answered for a particular firm. But if a firm plans, practices, and manages the PAI up to this point, it can manage this issue. The firm will understand the upsides and downsides of each of the issues because it has planned ahead. Knowing all of the pluses and minuses should make the decisions clear—not easy, but clear.

REFERENCE

1. J. Phillips, University of Georgia GMP Conference, March 1996.

7

The Validation of Pharmaceutical Processes

Robert A. Nash
St. John's University, Jamaica, New York

I. PRE–NEW DRUG APPLICATION APPROVAL INSPECTIONS

The Food and Drug Administration's (FDA's) pre-approval inspection program [1] is designed to provide a basis for determining the adequacy and accuracy of reported technical information in new drug application (NDA) and abbreviated NDA (ANDA) submissions with respect to the suitability of current Good Manufacturing Procedures (cGMP) product development, analytical laboratories, and manufacturing facilities.

Adequate preparation for an FDA pre-NDA approval inspection includes having the following documentation ready before the formal inspection:

1. Active drug substance development and validation report(s) including impurity profile and polymorphic forms
2. Pharmaceutical (dosage form) development report
3. Stability and clinical batch records and history, including phase III program
4. Data for active drug substance and key excipients used in the manufacture of clinical and biobatches
5. Bioequivalency report
6. Technology transfer report (from development to manufacturing)
7. Copy of NDA's Chemistry Manufacturing and Control (CMC) section, including information on suppliers and vendors
8. Copy of proposed production monograph and master batch record

9. Equipment validation report establishing installation qualification/ operational qualification (IQ/OQ)
10. Cleaning validation report
11. Analytical methods validation and computer systems validation reports
12. Process validation protocol for formal, three batch validation of production size batches

As can be seen from this list, validation plays a key role in pre-NDA approval inspections.

Agency policy during pre-approval inspections is to accept a process validation protocol based on the company's commitment to successfully complete three production-size validation batches before product launch. In some situations, either a prevalidation demonstration (process qualification) production-size batch is completed or the entire formal three-batch program is conducted.

This chapter addresses many of the validation issues key to successful product development, and thus essential to a successful pre-NDA approval inspection.

II. THE VALIDATION OF PHARMACEUTICAL PROCESSES

Process validation, a requirement of cGMP for finished pharmaceuticals (21 CFR 211), applies to the manufacturing of drug products during the process development stages as well as commercial production.

According to the FDA's guidelines on general principles of process validation [2], process validation is defined "as establishing documented evidence, which provides a high degree of assurance, that a specific process will consistently produce a product meeting its predetermined specifications and quality characteristics." The process for making a drug product consists of a series (flow diagram in logically defined steps) of unit operations (modules) that results in the manufacture of the finished clinical trial material and finished pharmaceuticals.

There is much confusion as to what process validation is and what constitutes process validation documentation. The term validation is generically used to cover the entire spectrum of cGMP concerns, most of which are essentially facility, equipment, component, method, and process qualification. Based on the process validation guidelines [2], the specific term should be reserved for the final stage(s) of the product and process development sequence. The essential or key steps or stages of a successfully completed development program are presented in Table 1.

The end of the development sequence that should be assigned to formal (three-batch) process validation derives from the fact that the specific exercise of

Table 1 Process Validation Is the Last
Step in the Procedure, Not the First Step

Developmental stage	Batch size
Product design	1X
Product characterization	
Product selection	
Process design	
Product optimization	10X
Process characterization	
Process optimization	
Process qualification	
Process qualification	100X
Process validation	
Process certification	
Process revalidation	100X to 1000X

process validation should be designed to succeed. Failure to conduct the formal process validation requirement assignment is often the result of incomplete or faulty understanding of process capability; in other words, what the process can and cannot do under a given set of operational requirements.

In a well-designed validation program, most of the effort should be spent on facilities, equipment, component, methods, and process qualification. In such a program, the formalized, final three-batch validation sequence provides only the necessary process validation documentation required by the FDA to show product reproducibility and a manufacturing process in a state of control. Such a strategy is consistent with FDA's pre-approval inspection program directive [1].

A. Process Validation Options

The guidelines on general principles of process validation [2] mention three options: prospective process validation (also called premarket validation), retrospective process validation, and revalidation. In actuality, there are four, if concurrent process validation is included—prospective process validation being the most important for an FDA pre-NDA approval inspection of a new chemical entity (NCE) or active pharmaceutical ingredient (API) in a dosage form or delivery system.

1. Prospective Validation

Prospective validation is conducted before the distribution of either a new product or an existing product made under a revised manufacturing process where such revisions may affect product specifications or quality characteristics (attributes). The prospective approach features critical step analysis, in which the unit operations are challenged during the process qualification stage to determine, using either "worst case" analysis or a fractional factorial design, critical process variables that may affect overall process performance. During formal, three-batch, prospective validation, critical process variables should be set within their operating ranges and should not exceed their upper and lower control limits during process operation. Output responses should be well within finished product specifications.

2. Retrospective Validation

Retrospective validation is recognized in both cGMP (21 CFR 211.110b) and the process validation guidelines [2]. It involves using the accumulated in-process production and final product testing and control (numerical) data to establish that the product and its manufacturing process are in a state of control. Valid in-process results should be consistent with the drug products final specifications and should be derived from previous acceptable process average and process variability estimates, where possible, and determined by the application of suitable statistical procedures, i.e., quality control charting, where appropriate.

The retrospective validation option is selected for established products whose manufacturing processes are considered to be stable and when, on the basis of economic considerations and resource limitations, prospective qualification and validation experimentation cannot be justified. Before undertaking either prospective or retrospective validation, the facilities, equipment, and subsystems used in connection with the manufacturing process must be qualified in conformance with cGMP requirements.

3. Concurrent Validation

Concurrent validation is studies that are conducted under a protocol during the course of normal production. The first three production-scale batches must be monitored as comprehensively as possible. The evaluation of the results is used in establishing the acceptance criteria and specifications of subsequent in-process control and final product testing. Some form of concurrent validation, using statistical process control techniques (quality control charting), may be used throughout the product manufacturing life cycle.

4. Revalidation

Revalidation is required to assure that changes in process and/or in the process environment, whether introduced intentionally or unintentionally, do not adversely affect product specifications and quality characteristics [2]. There should be a quality assurance system (change control) in place that requires revalidation whenever there are significant changes in formulation, equipment, process, and packaging that may impact on product and manufacturing process performance [3]. Furthermore, when a change is made in a raw material supplier, the drug product manufacturer should be made aware of subtle, potentially adverse differences in raw material characteristics that may adversely affect product and manufacturing process performance.

It is recommended that every requested change be reviewed by the validation or CMC committee. Such a committee should judge if a change is significant for revalidation or scale-up and post-approval changes (SUPAC) and then decide on a course of action to be taken. Conditions requiring revalidation study and documentation are listed as follows:

1. Change in a critical component (usually refers to active pharmaceutical ingredient, key excipient, or primary packaging)
2. Change or replacement in a critical piece of modular (capital) equipment
3. Significant change in processing conditions that may affect subsequent unit operations and product quality
4. Change in a facility and/or plant (usually location, site, or support systems)
5. Significant increase or decrease in batch size that affects the operation of modular equipment
6. Sequential batches that fail to meet product and process specifications

In some situations, process performance requalification studies may be required before undertaking specific revalidation assignments. With the exception of sterile products manufacture, periodic revalidation is not required at the present time. The performance and state of control of the product and its manufacturing process can be adequately covered during the annual product and process review. The FDA has issued an interim guidance document that addresses what constitutes major and minor formulations and manufacturing changes for immediate-release solid dosage forms (SUPAC-IR) [4]. Such documentation and others to follow should simplify manufacturing decisions about the need to revalidate.

III. VALIDATION MASTER PLAN

The creation of a master plan enables one to develop an overview of the validation effort. Such a plan should be created early in the drug development process and updated on a regular basis. This plan should be linked to the overall drug development plan. The plan lays out in a logical sequence the activities and/or key elements to be performed versus the approximate time schedule in a Gantt or Program Evaluation and Review Technique (PERT) chart format. Once generated, the master plan establishes the critical path against which progress can be monitored and linked to other drug development activities.

The validation program starts with the design and development of raw materials and components, and is then followed by the IQ/OQ of facilities, equipment, and systems, through performance and process qualification stages, and terminates in the protocol-driven, three-batch, formal process validation program undertaken before launch. Many of these activities move forward in series. However, by combining activities and elements in groups and moving in parallel, where possible, on independent tracks with respect to APIs, analytical methods development, facilities, equipment, support systems, and the drug product design and manufacturing process development itself, a great deal of time can be saved before the individual elements or groupings of activities come together before the formal process validation program. Such a Gantt chart format has been constructed and is shown in Figure 1.

The following three stages with respect to equipment qualification are sometimes referred to as Equipment Validation:

1. *IQ*: Procedures and documentation to show that all important aspects of the installation of either the facility, support system, or piece of modular equipment, having been properly calibrated, meet their design specifications and that the vendor's recommendations had been suitably considered.

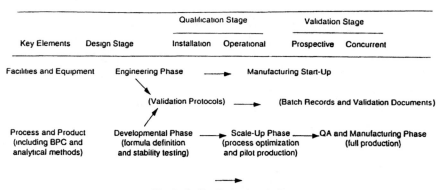

Figure 1   Validation progress Gantt chart.

2. *OQ*: Following IQ, procedures and documentation that showed the facility, support system, or piece of modular equipment performed as intended throughout all anticipated operating ranges under a suitable load
3. *Performance Qualification (PQ)*: Following IQ and OQ, actual demonstrations during the course of the validation program that showed the facility, support system, or piece of modular equipment performed according to a predefined protocol and achieved process reproducibility and product acceptability

IV. VALIDATION PROTOCOL AND REPORT

The following validation protocol and format for the completed validation report have been suggested in the Guidelines on the Validation of Manufacturing Processes [5]. The format for the validation report provides a useful template on previous reports for the FDA pre-NDA approval inspection.

1. Purpose (for the whole validation) and prerequisites
2. Presentation of the whole process and subprocesses, including flow diagram and critical step analysis
3. Validation protocol approvals
4. IQ and OQ, including blueprints or drawings
5. Qualification report(s)
   a. Subprocess 1
   b. Purpose
   c. Methods/procedures
   d. Sampling and testing procedures, release criteria
   e. Reporting function
   f. Calibration of test equipment used
   g. Test data
   h. Summary of results
   i. Approval and requalification procedure
   Subprocess 2 (repeat a through i) and so forth
6. Product qualification, test data from prevalidation batches
7. Product validation, test data from three formal validation batches
8. Evaluation and recommendations (include revalidation/requalification requirements)
9. Certification (approval)
10. Summary report with conclusions

The validation protocol and report may also include copies of the product stability report or its summary plus validation documentation concerning cleaning and analytical methods. It is prudent to add the cleaning and analytical methods documentation because they can be required by the FDA during the pre-approval inspection.

V. PILOT SCALE-UP AND TECHNOLOGY TRANSFER

The pilot-production program may be conducted either as a shared responsibility between the development laboratories and its appropriate manufacturing counterpart or as a process demonstration by a separate, designated pilot-plant or process development function. The decision of how to conduct pilot production in many cases depends on how the company is organized and the degree of cooperation that exists between the research and manufacturing operations. The stage of development is also a critical variable that needs to be taken into consideration. Supporting technology transfer documentation applies to both the specific process/system being qualified and validated and its testing standards and testing methods. The formal technology transfer is normally made from either the development laboratories or the process development pilot-plant to pharmaceutical production function just before launch.

In actuality, there are a number of technology transfer points and documents that take place as the prospective validation program proceeds through the various stages of product and process development. These stages of technology transfer in terms of scale-up are illustrated in Figure 2. The documentation from these stages is key to a successful pre-NDA approval inspection.

Solid pharmaceutical dosage forms (tablets and capsules) will be used to illustrate the various stages of product and process development. These principles and practices also apply in a general way to the development of liquid and semisolid pharmaceutical dosage forms (not discussed here). Sterile products manufactured for injectables and ophthalmic dosage forms are usually covered in separate monographs.

Elements of the validation concept should be incorporated during each of the various stages of the product and process development continuum. These stages have been summarized as follows:

Stage 0	Preformulation studies: bulk pharmaceutical chemicals
Stage I	Product design and development
Stage II	Preparation of clinical and bio-batches
Stage III	Process scale-up and evaluation
Stage IV	Formal process validation

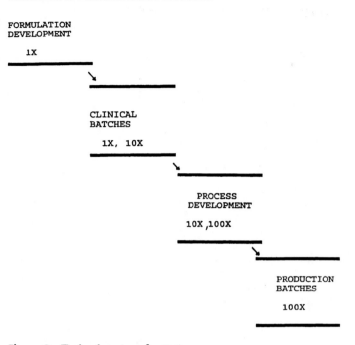

FORMULATION
DEVELOPMENT

1X

CLINICAL
BATCHES

1X, 10X

PROCESS
DEVELOPMENT

10X ,100X

PRODUCTION
BATCHES

100X

Figure 2 Technology transfer stages.

A. Preformulation Studies: Bulk Pharmaceutical Chemicals

Preformulation testing of the specific active pharmaceutical ingredient of interest and key excipients that will be used in the product design stage, alone and in binary combinations with the active drug substance, should be included as a preliminary first step in the product and process development sequence.

A simple checklist of items that one might consider when conducting preformulation studies with bulk pharmaceutical chemicals (both APIs and important or critical excipients) is provided in Table 2. Consideration of the items will facilitate the drug development process and FDA approval process.

Several factors must be kept in mind before preformulation studies are undertaken: (1) It is imperative that two-way technical communication between the manufacturers of the active drug substance (laboratory and plant) and the pharmaceutical product development laboratories be established. It should start early and be maintained throughout the product and process development life cycle. Such communication will ensure that the product is developed appropriately and thus enhance the chances of passing the pre-approval inspection in a

Table 2 Preformulation Studies: Bulk Pharmaceutical Chemicals

Active drug substance
  Key excipients
    Fillers/diluents
    Binders
    Disintegrants
    Glidants/lubricants
    • Chemical and physical compatibility
    • Minimum lot-to-lot variability in properties
    • Available worldwide from comparable suppliers

Properties for possible evaluation
  Aspect: Color, odor, taste, solubility
  Particle morphology, including DSC, TGA, x-ray
  Different particle size distribution and surface area
  Crystal and bulk density and compaction index
  Angle of repose and flowability index
  Spectrophotometry: UV, FTIR, NMR, OR
  Water content, LOD and moisture uptake
  Microbial limits and heavy metals
  HPLC assay and impurity profile

DSC, differential scanning calorimetry; TGA, thermal gravimetric analysis; UV, ultraviolet; FTIR, Fourier transformed infrared spectrometry; NMR, nuclear magnetic resonance; OR, optical rotation; LOD, loss on drying; HPLC, high-performance liquid chromatography.

timely manner. (2) In addition to potency, purity, and stability considerations of the active drug substance, Product Development is especially interested in the chemical and physical form (free acid or base, salts, esters, amides, polymorphs, solvates, particle size, and shape) of the active drug substance. Time spent early in the product development cycle in getting these particular factors established will often aid and/or simplify the subsequent product and process development program.

Not every item provided or listed in Table 2 must be tested or addressed. One or more items, however, in each of the main categories (aspect, particle morphology and size, compaction and flowability, water content, spectro-photometry and chromatography) should be studied and monitored throughout the product and process development program [6, 7].

Since key excipients are well established in most new product and process development programs, the same degree of preformulation scrutiny is often not required. Binary compatibility studies with the active drug substance, however, should be performed to study possible untoward interactions between the actives and such key excipients.

It should be kept in mind that small or minor changes in physical and possibly chemical properties upon intimate contact in binary studies with key excipients should not automatically rule out the use of a favored excipient without further critical testing.

B. Stage One: Product Design and Development

After successful preformulation studies, the active pharmaceutical ingredient is transferred to the formulations laboratory for preliminary product design and development studies. In most cases, the drug is admixed with an appropriate diluent/filler and glidant combination and filled with two-piece opaque hard-shell capsules for preliminary stability and subsequent phase I clinical studies versus matching placebo capsules [8].

On or about the same time, initial studies of a prototype tablet formulation should be started. The key steps in the product design and development sequence are outlined in Table 3. Although the work is conducted in the research or formulations laboratory using small-scale processing equipment, it is important to gain early experience with colorant systems that have been selected for the final finished tablet product. The use of color will aid in blend uniformity evaluation.

In addition to excipient screening and selection, it is important to gauge processing parameters that will be more fully explored during the future process scale-up phases. These processing factors include flowability, compaction and compressibility of powder and granules, content uniformity of powder and granule blends and finished tablets, moisture uptake, in vitro dissolution release profiles, and subsequent full-scale stability testing. Product that is used in human clinical trials will, of course, conform to good laboratory, good clinical, and GMP requirements [1, 9].

C. Stage Two: Process Development, Pilot-Laboratory (Clinical)

After the (1X) "go" laboratory batch has been determined to be both physically and chemically stable based on accelerated, elevated temperature testing (i.e., 1 month at 45°C or 3 months at 40°C or 40°C/80% relative humidity), the next step (stage 2) is to scale the product and its process to (10X) pilot-laboratory size batch(es). The (10X) pilot-laboratory size batch represents the first replicated scale-up of the designated formula. The size of the pilot-laboratory batch will usually range between 10 and 100 kg, 10 and 100 L, or 10,000 and 100,000 units. These pilot-laboratory batches are often used in clinical trials and bioequivalency

Table 3 Stage One: Product Design, 1X Laboratory Scale (1–10 kg)

Hard shell capsule (phase I clinical trials) followed by prototype tablet dosage form
Direct compression vs. wet granulation
Maximize chemical and physical stability
Minimize product and process costs
  • Product design
  • Product characterization
  • Product selection
  • Process design
Excipients selected from the following lists:
  Binder/diluent/disintegrant
    Alginates, calcium phosphate, cellulose and derivatives, dextrates, gelatin, povidone
    and derivatives, starch and derivatives, sorbitol, sucrose and derivatives.
  Glidant/lubricant
    Colloidal silicon dioxide, hydrogenated vegetable oil, mineral oil, PEGs, silica gel,
    sodium lauryl sulfate, stearates, talc.

studies. According to the FDA, the minimum requirement for a bio-batch is 100,000 units [10].

The pilot-laboratory batches are usually prepared in small pilot equipment within a designated cGMP-approved facility. The number and size of these pilot-laboratory batches may vary in response to one or more of the following factors: (1) equipment availability; (2) active pharmaceutical ingredient availability; (3) cost of raw materials; and (4) inventory requirements for both clinical and nonclinical studies.

Process development (process qualification) or process capability studies are normally started in this important second stage of the scale-up sequence. The scope of stage two (process development) is presented in Table 4 and consists essentially of product optimization and process characterization studies.

Unit operations are selected for the development of either a tablet (coated or noncoated) or capsule (hard shell or soft gel) process [11]. Unit operations that are considered to be critical are determined through an analysis of the process variables and their respective measured responses in each unit operation (Table 5) [12–14].

To get a handle on the critical control parameters and their unit operation, constraint analysis techniques [15] followed by fractional factorial designs (Table 6) are used to challenge the tentative control limits (so-called worst case analysis) established for the process at this intermediate stage. Time and effort spent to qualify the process at the 10X stage will often simplify the work that follows during stages three and four.

Table 4 Stage Two: Process Development: 10X Pilot-Laboratory, Clinical[a] (10–100 kg)

First product and process scale-up experience in a GMP facility
  Product optimization
    Establish formula rationale and boundary conditions for active and excipients
  Process characterization
    Define unit operations, process variables, and response parameters
    Define critical process variables and response parameters using simple experimental
      designs
    Establish provisional control limits for critical process variables and their response
      parameters based on process replication
  Maintain product stability
Unit operations for solid dosage form development include:
  Granulation
  Drying
  Sizing
  Blending/mixing
  Encapsulation/tablet compression
  Coating

[a]Bio-batch should be at least 100,000 units.

von Doehren et al. [13] and Chowhan [16] have written articles on the various stages of solid dosage form process development as it relates to technology transfer and process validation. Their respective approaches to the topic have been integrated and added to (Tables 3–5).

Fahrner [17], in his article "New Role for Pilot Plants in Product Development," raises the following issues:

1. There is too much preliminary or applied research and not enough time is devoted to the proper development of the process.
2. There is often a lack of a suitable manufacturing strategy during the early phases of the program, which often results in poorly planned technology transfer and an inappropriate division of responsibility with respect to the overall program.
3. Most laboratory processes are rarely scaleable, since piloting is a scaled-down version of manufacturing, not a scaled-up version of the laboratory batch.

Addressing these issues will minimize the chance of encountering problems and, therefore, maximize the chances for developing a validated process. Fahrner makes the case for a separate pilot facility (process development function) to bridge the communication gap between R&D and production.

Table 5 Control Parameters for Consideration in Solid Dosage Form Development

Unit operation	Process variables (X's)	Measured responses (Y's)
Granulation (power type)	Load Speed (main/chopper) Liquid addition rate Granulation time	Power consumption
Drying	Load Inlet temperature Air flow rate Drying time	Moisture content Bulk density
Sizing (screening)	Load Screen size Speed Feed rate	Particle size distribution Bulk density
Blending (mixing)	Load Speed Mixing time	Blend uniformity
Encapsulation	Fill volume Tamper setting Speed Glidant (type and amount)	Capsule weight Moisture content Dissolution Content uniformity Potency
Tablet compression	Press speed Feed rate Precompression force Compression force	Tablet weight Moisture content Hardness/friability Thickness Dissolution/disintegration Content uniformity Potency
Coating (film type)	Load Pan speed Spray rate Air flow	Weight gain

[a]Seven to 23 possible variables; 11 to 16 possible responses.

Table 6 New Fractional Factorial Design for Development[a]

	Seven Variables — Eight Trials Key Variables[a]							
Trials	X_1	X_2	X_3	X_4	X_5	X_6	X_7	Sums
1	−	−	−	−	−	−	−	0/7
2	−	−	−	+	−	−	−	1/6
3	−	−	+	−	−	+	−	2/5
4	+	+	−	−	+	−	−	3/4
5	+	+	−	−	−	+	+	4/3
6	+	−	+	+	+	−	+	5/2
7	−	+	+	+	+	+	+	6/1
8	+	+	+	+	+	+	+	7/0
Sums	4/4	4/4	4/4	4/4	4/4	4/4	4/4	28/28

[a]Key variables are randomly assigned "X_{no}" value.
Adapted from C. D. Hendrix, What every technologist should know about experimental design, Chemtech (March 1979).

D. Stage Three: Pilot Program

The technology transfer of the product and process from the traditional product development function to either a separate process development (pilot plant) function or production itself is normally conducted at the (100X) pilot-production batch stage (Table 7). The creation of a separate pilot plant or Process Development unit has been favored in recent years because this particular organizational structure is ideally suited to conduct key PQ and/or process validation studies in a timely manner [18, 19].

The objective of the pilot-production batch is to scale the product and its process by another order of magnitude (100X). For most solid dosage forms, it represents a full production scale batch in standard production equipment. The technology transfer documents should include the technical package normally required for pre-approval inspection:

1. Preformulation information
2. Product development report
3. Product stability report
4. Analytical methods report
5. Proposed manufacturing formula manufacturing instruction, in-process and final product specifications at the 100X batch size.

The objectives of pre-validation trials at stage three (100X Pilot-Production) are to qualify and optimize the process in full-scale production equipment and facilities.

Table 7 Stage Three: Process Scale-Up and Evaluation: 100X Pilot-Production
Batch(es) (100–1000 kg)

Full-scale production batch
For possible clinical/future commercial use
Evaluate critical process parameters
    Product and process is scaled to another order of magnitude (100X)
Process optimization
    Mixing/blending times
    Drying times
    Milling operations
    Press speed/compression force
    Encapsulation speed/tamping settings
    Speed/air flow/spray settings/temperature
Process qualification (prevalidation batch(es))
    Determine process capability
    Challenge in-process control limits
Maintain product stability

Rushing through the first (100X) pilot-production batch to get on with formal
validation should be discouraged despite the pressure to get to market quickly.
Small problems that often arise during (100X) scale-up should be addressed
immediately and not ignored. Such problems are often best addressed by returning
to the laboratories (1X and/or 10X) for supplemental process characterization and
qualification studies.

Many companies, however, go directly to three-batch formal validation
without stage three prevalidation work and often complete formal trials before
pre-approval inspection. The downside of this alternative strategy is that finished
production batches often sit in the warehouse beyond their approval expiry dating
period. But it is a risk many pharmaceutical companies take in the hopes of
increasing their chances of passing the FDA pre-NDA approval inspection in a
timely manner.

There is no ideal way of completing the pilot scale-up and validation
sequence. Many companies depend on their prior experience with related products
and processes in making a choice of strategies.

E. Stage Four: Formal Process Validation

In the normal course of events and after a successful completed pre-approval
inspection, formal, three-batch process validation will be conducted in accordance

with the protocol approved during the pre-approval inspection. The primary objective of the formal process validation exercise is to establish process reproducibility and consistency. Such validation must be completed before entering the product into interstate commerce after FDA approval. The program is not designed to challenge upper and lower control units (so-called worst case analysis) of critical process variables. Such upper and lower control limit challenging is normally conducted during the stage two (10X size) process characterization, optimization, and qualification program using suitable and reasonable experimental designs (Table 6).

The documentation to be established before, during, and after formal process validation is outlined in Table 8. The protocols and the subsequent formal validation studies are designed to establish uniformity among the three batches with respect to granulation, mixing or blending, finished tablet, and finished capsule stage [1, 2, 10]. In that respect, the following test data and result are used to show process reproducibility and consistency among validation batches:

1. Particle or granule size distribution
2. Bulk density
3. Moisture content
4. Hardness
5. Thickness
6. Friability

Table 8   Stage Four: Formal Process Validation, 100X Production Batches

Complete product development program and report
Prepare protocol for prospective process validation
Complete pre-approval inspection requirements
   Conduct 3-batch formal process validation
   Establish reproducibility for mixing/blending and compression or encapsulation
     operations
Establish, process, documentation
   Preformulation report
   Analytical methods validation report
   IQ/OQ and cleaning validation reports
   Formula development report
   Process feasibility report
   Manufacturing bioequivalency report
   Product development report
   Process validation protocol
   Process validation report
   Product stability report

7. Weight uniformity
8. Potency uniformity
9. Disintegration/dissolution profile
10. Product stability

Not every one of the 10 listed items or categories has to be addressed or followed both during in-process and final product testing. Nevertheless, sufficient testing must be conducted to establish process reproducibility and to demonstrate, with a high degree of certainty, that the product and process are in a state of control.

Whenever possible, formal validation studies should continue through packaging and labeling operations (in whole or in part), so that machinability and stability of the finished product can be established and documented in the primary container-closure system.

1. Change Control

Procedures with respect to establishing change control should be in place before, during, and after the completion of the formal validation program. A change control system maintains a sense of functionality as the process evolves, and also provides the necessary documentation trail that ensures that the process continues in a validated, operational state even when small noncritical adjustments and changes have been made to the process.

Such minor, noncritical changes in materials, methods, and machines should be reviewed by the validation or CMC committee (Development, Engineering, Production, and Quality Assurance/Quality Control) to assure all that process integrity and process comparability have been maintained and documented before the specific change that has been requested can be approved by the head of the Quality Control Unit.

The change control system, based on an approved standard operating procedure (SOP), takes on added importance as the vehicle or instrument through which innovation and process improvements can be made more easily and more flexible without prior formal review on the part of the NDA and ANDA reviewing function of the FDA. If more of the supplemental procedures with respect to the Chemistry and Manufacturing Control sections of NDAs and ANDAs are covered through annual SUPAC review documentation procedures, with appropriate safeguards, process validation will become more pro-innovative [20–22].

VI. CLEANING VALIDATION

According to section 211.67 Equipment Cleaning and Maintenance of cGMP regulations [3], equipment and utensils should be cleaned, maintained, and sanitized at appropriate intervals to prevent malfunction or contamination that would alter the safety, identity, strength, quality, or purity of the drug product. This includes materials used in clinical trials as well as the commercial drug product. Written procedures should be established and followed for cleaning and maintenance of equipment in both product development laboratories and manufacturing facilities. These procedures should include, but are not limited to, the following:

1. Assignment of responsibility for cleaning and maintaining equipment
2. Maintenance and cleaning schedules and sanitizing schedules where appropriate
3. Description in sufficient detail of methods, equipment, and material used in cleaning and maintenance operations, and the methods of disassembling and reassembling equipment as necessary to ensure proper cleaning and maintenance
4. Removal or obliteration of previous batch identification
5. Protecting of clean equipment from contamination before use
6. Inspection of equipment for cleanliness immediately before use

Records should be kept of maintenance, cleaning, sanitizing, and inspection. The FDA may ask for these records during the course of the pre-approval inspection.

The objective of cleaning validation of equipment and utensils is to reduce the residues of one product below established limits so that the residue of the previous product does not affect the quality and safety of the subsequent product manufactured in the same equipment.

According to section 211.63 Equipment Design, Size and Location of cGMP regulations [3], equipment used in the manufacture, processing, packing, or holding of a drug product shall be of appropriate design and adequate size and suitability located to facilitate operations for its intended use and for its cleaning and maintenance.

Some of the equipment design considerations include type of surface to be cleaned (stainless steel, glass, plastic), use of disposables or dedicated equipment and utensils (bags, filters, etc.), use of stationary equipment (tanks, mixers, centrifuges, presses, etc.), use of special features (clean-in-place systems, steam-in-place systems), and identifying the difficult-to-clean locations on the equipment (so-called "hot spots" and/or critical sites).

The specific cleaning procedure should define the amounts and the specific type of cleaning agents and/or solvents used. The cleaning procedure should give full details as to what is to be cleaned and how it is to be cleaned. The cleaning method should focus on worse-case conditions, such as higher strength, least-soluble, most difficult to clean formulations. Cleaning procedures should identify time between processing and cleaning, cleaning sequence, equipment dismantling procedure, the need for visual inspection, and provisions for documentation.

The choice of a particular analytical method high-performance liquid chromatography (HPLC), thin-layer chromatography (TLC), spectrophotometric, total organic carbon, pH, conductivity, gravimetric, etc.) and sampling technique chosen (direct surface by swabs and gauze or by rinsing) will depend on the residue limit to be established based on the sampling site, type of residue sought, and equipment configuration (critical sites vs large surface area) consideration. The analytical and sampling methods should be challenged in terms of specificity, sensitivity, and recovery.

The established residue limits must be practical, achievable, and verifiable, and they must assure safety. The potency of the selected drug, presence of degradation products, cleaning agents, and microorganisms should be taken into consideration.

The following residue limits have been suggested: not more than (NMT) 10 ppm; NMT, 0.001. The dose of any product will appear in the maximum daily dose of another product, and no physical or chemical residue will be visible on the equipment after cleaning procedures have been performed.

VII. ANALYTICAL METHODS VALIDATION

Analytical methods go to the heart of a validated process for drug product manufacture. More time and resources are spent in generating quality analytical data (numbers) before, during, and after pre-approval inspections than any other aspect of the pharmaceutical process validation program. Simply stated, analytical methods answer two basic questions for us: What is it? and How much is present in the specific entity undergoing testing?

Analytical methods are used in the testing of the following product and processing elements:

1. Active pharmaceutical ingredients
2. Individual inert excipients
3. Impurities for products, actives, and inerts
4. Residues from previously used materials and operations
5. In-process compositions and blends
6. Final, finished dosage forms before release

Such analytical data are required in each and every stage of the development and manufacturing processing life cycle. The stages include preformulation studies, formulation development, batches for clinical study, process development and scale-up, formal process validation, routine production, change control, revalidation, and stability testing throughout the entire program.

Since a typical analytical method (usually chromatographic) combines columns, pumps, heaters, detectors, controllers, samplers, sensors, recorders, computers, reagents, standards, and operators, it is considered to be a system. As such, and like a process for the manufacture of a specific product, it requires validation. The elements listed above from columns through operators (or analytical chemists) all require qualification before formal, protocol-driven validation.

Once the basics of the system have been qualified, information supporting the suitability of the analytical method should be established beyond a reasonable degree of certainty. Such data should include the accuracy, precision, and linearity over the range of interest, i.e., 80% to 120% of label potency. Data demonstrating the specificity, sensitivity, ruggedness of the method and the limits for degradation products and/or impurities should be included. Furthermore, degradation products and impurities should be adequately identified and characterized. Data demonstrating recovery of actives, and lack of interference from other components, reagents, and standards should be demonstrated. Data characterizing day-to-day, laboratory-to-laboratory, analyst-to-analyst, and column-to-column variability should be developed to supplement reproducibility and ruggedness information. The validated analytical method should be stability indicating. Recognition by an official compendium will often simplify the requirements listed above.

Biological assay methods as well as the identification and analysis of microorganisms should be held to similar but reasonable standards in conformance with the limitation of biological testing.

VIII. COMPUTER SYSTEM VALIDATION

Pharmaceutical dosage form and medical device manufacturers are responsible for the validation of all custom-designed computer systems, especially those used in connection with automated processes.

Each computer system should be separately defined and inventoried, especially those that are used to control specified manufacturing processes and operations. Computer systems are important extensions of the processes that they are designed to control and/or monitor. The use of computers, automation devices, and programmable logic controllers (PLCs) in the production and control of drug products is on the rise.

A computer system consists of hardware, i.e., physical and calibration devices, sensors, input/output (I/O) devices, transducers, or equipment, and its companion software that is used to generate records, instructions, and/or data. Source codes and supporting software documentation used in drug process control is considered to be part of the master production and control records under cGMP interpretation.

It is important to separate computer systems into their varied and appropriate categories:

1. Computer integrated manufacturing (CIM)
2. Analytical instrumentation and automated laboratory practices (GALPs)
3. Computer controlled, electronic signature systems
4. Computer integrated packaging operations
5. Laboratory information management systems (LIMS)
6. Computer systems for good clinical practice (GCP)
7. Computer assisted medical devices

All of the categories listed above require qualification and validation documentation.

With respect to pharmaceutical process development and manufacturing operations, the highest priority should be given to computer integrated manufacturing. Total process automation and companion CIM operations should not be initiated until sufficient prospective and concurrent validation studies have been successfully completed. The rush to automation should be discouraged until process capability information has been established for all critical and most manual unit operations.

Because the validation of a computer hardware/software system does not differ in principle from the validation of pharmaceutical processes and analytical methods, the basic approach to validation should be familiar:

Hardware Validation
1. Installation and component qualification in addition to vendor support
2. Operational qualification and modular testing
3. Performance qualification in conjunction with functional software testing
4. Operational reproducibility
5. Reconfiguration and change control as required

Software Validation
1. Functional testing where defined inputs produce outputs that meet expectations and/or specifications
2. Structural testing that includes a thorough examination of source codes, database designs, programming standards, control methods, and support documentation
3. Quality assurance program that includes alternate plans, contingency practices, record retrieval, and security practices

A flow diagram for the validation of a new and existing computer system is presented in Figure 3. The information was developed by the PhRMA's Computer System Validation Committee in the early 1990s.

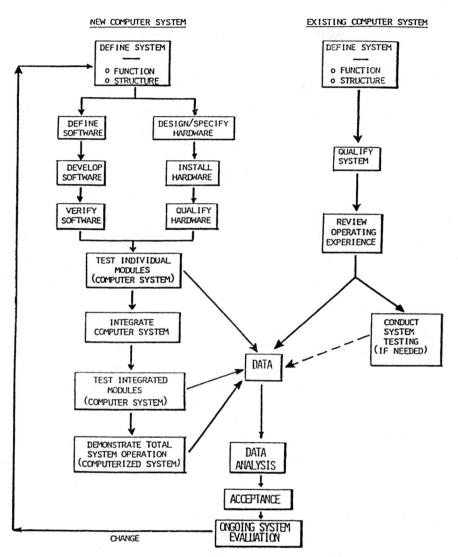

Figure 3 Validation life cycle approach. [From Joseph M. George, Real-life experiences in computer system validation. *Pharm. Technol.* 18(11), 1994.]

IX. CONCLUSIONS

The advent of FDA pre-NDA approval inspections added a new step in the new drug approval process: the review of GMP compliance and the accuracy and adequacy of the data included in the NDA submission by the FDA field force. The FDA field investigators examine many facets of the product development work during the course of the investigation. One of the most important areas routinely addressed by the FDA during the inspection is validation. This chapter has covered how to approach validation during the course of the new product development cycle. Validation activities should be with the development of the master validation plan early in the product development life cycle. Prefacing and documenting the appropriate validation work over the entire drug development life cycle will greatly enhance the chances of passing the pre-approval inspection.

REFERENCES

1. FDA, *Pre-Approval Inspection/Investigations Guidance Manual, 7346.832*, 1990.
2. FDA, *Guideline on General Principles of Process Validation*, FDA, Rockville, MD, 1987.
3. Fed. Reg. 43(190), *Human and Veterinary Drugs, Current Good Manufacturing Practice in Manufacturing, Processing, Packing or Holding*, 1978, pp. 45014–45089.
4. L. J. Lucisano, R. M. Franz, FDA proposed guidance for CM and C changes: a review and industrial perspective, *Pharm. Technol* 19:30–40 (1995).
5. WHO, *Good Manufacturing Practices for Pharmaceutical Products—Guidelines on the Validation of Manufacturing Processes*, Geneva, 1993.
6. J. P. Skelly, et al., Scaleup of immediate release oral solid dosage forms. *Pharm. Res.* 10:313–316 (1993).
7. J. P. Skelly, et al., Scaleup of oral extended-release dosage forms, *Pharm. Res.* 10:1800–1804 (1993).
8. S. Bolton, Process validation for hard gelatin capsules, *Drug Cosm. Ind.* 134:42–48, 85–87 (1984).
9. H. L. Avallone, Development and scaleup of pharmaceuticals, *Pharm. Eng.* 10:38–41 (1990).
10. FDA, *Guide to Inspections of Oral Solid Dosage Forms Pre/Post Approval Issues for Development and Validation*, 1994.
11. I. R. Berry, Process validation for soft gelatin capsules, *Drug Cosm. Ind.* 134:26–35 (1984).
12. R. A. Nash, Process validation for solid dosage forms, *Pharm. Technol.* 3:105–107 (1979).
13. P. J. von Doehren, F. St. John Forbes, and C. D. Shively, An Approach to the Characterization and Technology Transfer of Solid Dosage Form Processes, *Pharm. Technol.* 6:139–156 (1982).

14. *Validation in Practice* (H. Sucker, ed.), Wissenschaftliche Verlagsegesellschaft GmbH, Stuttgart, 1983.
15. *Pharmaceutical Process Validation, Second Edition, Revised and Expanded,* (I. R. Berry and R. A. Nash, eds.) Marcel Dekker, New York, 1993.
16. Z. T. Chowhan, Development of a new drug substance into a compact tablet, *Pharm. Technol.* 16:58–67 (1992).
17. R. Fahrner, New role for pilot plants in product development, *Biopharm* 6:34–37 (1993).
18. H. L. Avallone and P. D'Eramo, Scaleup and validation of ANDA/NDA products, *Pharm. Eng.* 12:36–39 (1992).
19. G. Bala, An integrated approach to process validation, *Pharm. Eng.* 14:57–64 (1994).
20. K. G. Chapman, A history of validation in the United States part I, *Pharm. Technol.* 15:82–96 (1991).
21. J. Akers, Simplifying and improving process validation, *J. Parenteral Sci. Technol.* 47:281–284 (1993).
22. K. Tomamichel, et al., Pharmaceutical quality assurance: basic of validation, *Swiss Pharmacol.* 16:13–23 (1994).

BIBLIOGRAPHY

1. Validation of manufacturing processes, Fourth European Seminar on Quality Control, Geneva, Switzerland, September 25, 1980.
2. *Validation in Practice* (H. Sucker, ed.) Wissenschaftliche Verlagsegesellschaft GmbH, Stuttgart, 1983.
3. *Pharmaceutical Process Validation* (B. T. Loftus and R. A. Nash, eds.) Marcel Dekker, New York, 1984, 1993.
4. *Validation of Aseptic Pharmaceutical Processes* (F. J. Carleton and J. P. Agalloco, eds.) Marcel Dekker, New York, 1986.
5. *Statistical Design and Analysis in Pharmaceutical Science, Validation, Process Controls and Stability* (S-C Chow and J-P Liu, eds.) Marcel Dekker, New York, 1995.

8

Documentation Standards for Pre-Approval Inspections

Richard M. Justice, Jr.
Eli Lilly and Company, Indianapolis, Indiana

I. INTRODUCTION

The research and development process for new drug therapies is spread over many years, at great cost, with only a small portion of the chemicals entering clinical trials ever being approved for the market. A 1991 publication of the *Journal of Health Economics* reported the estimate of the average cost of new drug development. This estimate was based on a confidential survey of 12 U.S.-owned firms and estimated the average cost of new drug development to be $231 million calculated in 1987 dollars. The report also indicated that the average time for a new chemical entity (NCE) to pass through all of the phases of development from synthesis to clinical trial to market approval extended nearly 12 years [1].

The pre-approval inspection (PAI) program was introduced by the Food and Drug Administration (FDA) during the first quarter of 1990. This inspection was implemented to verify the accuracy and adequacy of the data that is submitted to the agency in the drug application. Failure of a PAI results in a delay in approval of new drugs, thus prolonging the time it takes to bring new treatments to the patient.

Each year, the FDA Office of Compliance publishes a list of reasons for withholding the approval of a new drug application (NDA) and abbreviated new drug application (ANDA). Every year the list provides examples of inadequate or inappropriate documentation practices, e.g., the incorrect contract laboratory was identified in the application, the incorrect laboratory analysis was listed in the application, raw data were missing, there is a lack of production batch records and component records, and biobatch records are not reconcilable.

Because of the high cost, high risk, and long development time lines, it is imperative that the data that support the approval of NDAs and ANDAs are rapidly available to the FDA during an inspection. These data, which were generated during the development process, should be properly recorded to ensure passing the PAI. Failure to provide the proper data and documentation during a PAI will result in a recommendation of nonapproval of the application—a very costly problem.

The objective of this chapter is to provide guidance concerning documentation practices to be focused on during the drug development process from prospective and retrospective approaches, which will greatly improve the probability of a successful PAI. Specific discussions will cover (1) the FDA's expectations for documents to be produced or to be examined during the PAI; (2) what actions one should take to meet the FDA's expectations with regard to proper documentation; (3) a comparison of prospective and retrospective documentation practices; and (4) the consequences of poor documentation practices.

II. FDA DOCUMENTATION REQUIREMENTS

A. Expectations of Document to Be Reviewed

The FDA has given guidance that all drugs are to be produced in compliance with current Good Manufacturing Practices (cGMP). The regulations governing the manufacture of drug products are found in Parts 210 and 211 of 21 Code of Federal Regulations (CFR). The agency clarified its position on drugs that are produced for clinical trials in humans or animals in the 1991 *Guideline on the Preparation of Investigational New Drug Products (Human and Animal)*. In that guideline, the FDA stated that it also expects clinical trial materials to be produced in compliance with the cGMPs.

During the early 1990s, the FDA and the pharmaceutical industry held several meetings throughout the United States to clarify issues that were raised concerning the conduct of the PAI. During an Industry Exchange Meeting held in Chicago in November 1991, a concern was raised regarding the age of laboratory data, manufacturing records, and the state of documentation practices for investigational drugs that were manufactured many years prior.

The agency responded:

The age and location of the data are not the most significant issues. We expect the data to be reviewable and contained in original documents. The data must support or justify the manufacturing process and the decision that the process will perform properly. Regardless of the age of the data and its location, one must be able to discern the reason for the decision that the process performs consistently [2].

When asked if the agency was retroactively applying the PAI regulations, the agency replied: "The regulations have not changed in this respect. The only thing that has changed is that the agency is now auditing the data that are being submitted with the application" [2]. Therefore, even though the agency recognizes that there are differences between manufacturing investigational products and manufacturing commercial products, its expectations for documentation are the same: they must be accurate, adequate, and available.

1. Data Accuracy

On September 10, 1991, the FDA issued a policy concerning fraud, untrue statements of material facts, and other activities (56 Federal Register 46191). The policy states that actions on the part of the applicant, applicant's employees, or applicant's agents that subvert the integrity of an FDA review process through acts such as submitting fraudulent applications, making untrue statements of material facts, or giving or promising bribes or illegal gratuities, may call into question the accuracy or integrity of some or all of the applicant's submissions to the FDA.

This policy has become to be known as the Applications Integrity Policy. The policy applies to new and abbreviated human and animal drug approval, biological product and establishment licenses, medical device premarket approvals, premarket notifications, and classification petitions. The policy also applies to food additive petitions and color additive petitions.

In the event that the integrity of the data in an application is questioned, the FDA will cease all scientific review activities until the agency conducts a validity assessment of the data in the submission. The applicant company is expected to complete certain corrective actions. After the applicant's internal audit, the FDA intends to conduct another assessment of the corrections made by the applicant. Corrective actions that are to be taken by the company are:

1. Cooperating fully with the FDA and other federal investigations looking to the cause, scope, and effects of any wrongful doing
2. Identifying individuals who were or may have been associated with wrongful acts, and removing them from any substantive authority on matters under FDA jurisdiction; in effect, this amounts to FDA-mandated company-initiated debarment

3. Conducting an internal review, preferably involving an outside consultant team, to identify any wrongful acts associated with applications, including discrepancies between manufacturing conditions identified in approved applications and manufacturing conditions occurring during actual production; reports generated by this review must be given to the FDA

4. Providing a written commitment, ordinarily in the form of a Consent Decree or agreement signed by the president, chief executive officer, or other official most responsible for the applicant's operations, to develop and implement a corrective action operating plan to prevent future instances of wrongful acts

It is clear that the FDA will audit the accuracy of the data that have been submitted in the NDA or ANDA. The agency has given specific guidelines to its inspection team, and to the pharmaceutical industry, stating that data accuracy will be checked during the PAI [3].

The FDA is requiring the industry to provide documented evidence that the firm knows what it is manufacturing, that the firm knows how to manufacture the new product, and that the firm can provide documentation to show that it has not jeopardized the identity, strength, purity, or quality of the new product. Therefore, it is critical that the data generated during the development process be of unquestionable integrity. The FDA's expectations for data integrity is reasonable. This is nothing more than good science.

The reliability of the data that are submitted to the FDA is crucial since it is the basis on which the FDA will determine if the applicant is capable of producing a safe and, in some instances, an efficacious drug. For NDAs, both safety and efficacy need to be demonstrated. For ANDAs, however, it is not necessary to prove efficacy since the efficacy of the drug product has already been demonstrated. If the FDA determines that the criteria for approval cannot be met due to questions regarding the accuracy of submitted data, the FDA will not approve the application.

Section III discusses actions one should take to ensure that data in the application are documented with accuracy and integrity.

2. Data Adequacy

The following is a familiar saying of many FDA inspectors: "If it wasn't written down, it never happened." The issue of having adequate data can be discussed from two different vantage points. First, one needs to consider the ability to supply the agency sufficient data that demonstrate that the company has adequate control to manufacture, process, package, and test the new drug product. Second, one needs to consider being able to supply the required documentation that will be requested during the PAI that relates to method validation and forensic samples.

During the PAI, the inspection team is required to examine documentation that demonstrates adequate control to manufacture, process, package, and test the new drug product. The FDA *Compliance Program Guidance Manual 7346.832, Pre-Approval Inspections/Investigations*, lists some of the documents which may be reviewed, including the following:

1. Production records of batches related to clinical trial materials used to demonstrate bioavailability or bioequivalence; these clinical trial batches could have been used in early clinical studies
2. Batch records that are submitted in the application that demonstrate that the proposed production process is the process that was used to manufacture the bioavailability, bioequivalency, or stability batches
3. Development notebooks that contain data on bioavailability, bioequivalency, or stability of the new drug product
4. Inventory records and/or receiving records of drug substance purchases
5. Analytical laboratory notebooks and logs

The FDA requires the following documentation to be available for forensic samples:

1. A copy of the batch production record or the development manufacturing record
2. A copy of the approved testing method if other than United States Pharmacopeia (USP); if the method is a USP method, one must identify the edition and supplement that was used for testing
3. A supplier's certificate of analysis for specific batches of each active and inactive collected
4. Reports on any test performed by the firm on active ingredients, such as methods, spectra, chromatograms, and charts
5. Analytical reports of the applicant's analysis of their product and corresponding innovator product
6. A copy of the reports received by the applicant from all biotesting facilities for all in vitro tests performed on the product covered by the ANDA

The submission of method validation/verification samples is required under 21 CFR 314.50. The FDA requires the following documentation to be available for validation/verification samples:

1. Analytical methodology for the method being validated
2. Any reports of analyses performed by the firm on the product lot
3. Spectra, chromatograms, and charts

3. Data Availability

The concept of "readily available" was established in the 21 CFR 211.80 (C). The cGMP requirement states that records that are covered under Subpart J of 21

CFR 211.80 should be readily available for authorized inspection. Records that are covered under Subpart J include production, control, or distribution records, i.e., the type of documents that will be reviewed during the PAI.

Although the term "readily available" is vague, general experience indicates that the retrieval of any record that takes more than 60 minutes is excessive. Under many circumstances, this time period would be more than adequate; however, one must consider the problems that may arise in global operations. Documents in these facilities are separated by time and space, i.e., they may be located in another country that has a 7 to 15-hour difference in time zone. A strategy for addressing this issue is discussed in Section III.

4. English Language

In an age of multinational, international, and transnational corporations, the pharmaceutical industry has found itself manufacturing, processing, packaging, and testing the investigational new drug product and conducting clinical trials in non-English–speaking areas of the world. The same is true for the commercial manufacture of the active pharmaceutical ingredient (API), as well as the commercial manufacture of the drug product.

It is a requirement under 21 CFR 312.23 (C) that a sponsor submit an accurate and complete English translation of each part of the Investigational New Drug (IND) application that is not in English. The same requirement is true for NDAs under 21 CFR 314.50 paragraph (G) [2].

Therefore, it is essential that sufficient time is allotted for the translation of all of the documents that are discussed in this chapter.

B. Documents to Be Reviewed

It is the responsibility of the FDA Office of Compliance to ascertain whether a company can manufacture, process, package, and test a drug product while protecting the identity, strength, purity, and quality of the product. One method of determining that a company is in control of its manufacturing processes is the review of documents that are related to the process of interest.

As was discussed earlier, the FDA has expectations that certain documentation will be available to be examined during the PAI. Some of these expectations have been delineated in guidance documents and compliance programs, while others have been deemed important to facilitate the PAI by virtue of experience. The following is a discussion of documentation that should be made available during the PAI. Section III deals with how these documents should be prepared for the PAI.

1. Batch Record

The batch record is all of the information that comprises the production history of a particular drug product, Type A Medicated Article, API, or manufactured intermediate. Further definition of the batch record is given in 21 CFR 211.188. The batch record should contain the following:

1. Dates of manufacture
2. Identity of individual major equipment and lines used
3. Specific identification of each batch of component or in-process material used
4. Weights and measures of components used in the course of processing
5. In-process and laboratory control results
6. Inspection of the packaging and labeling area before and after use
7. A statement of the actual yield and a statement of the percentage of theoretical yield at appropriate phases of processing
8. Complete labeling control records, including specimens or copies of all labeling used
9. Description of drug product containers and closures
10. Any sampling performed
11. Identification of the persons performing and directly supervising or checking each significant step in the operation
12. Any deviation report resulting from an investigation made according to 21 CFR 211.192
13. Results of examinations made in accordance with 21 CFR 211.134 (packaging and labeling inspections)

2. Change Control

Change control is the procedural system through which changes are reviewed, justified, documented, approved, and implemented in conformance with regulatory and corporate requirements. Document that should be made available are:

1. *Change Control Summary*: This is a summary of all changes made to date that affect the manufacturing process being considered for approval.
2. *Change Control Reports*: These are individual reports that are written to review, justify, approve, and implement specific changes that affect the manufacturing process being considered for approval. These documents may include any change control reports for facilities, manufacturing processes, cleaning processes, or analytical laboratory methods that are related to the NDA/ANDA process being submitted.

Because of the nature of development activities and responsibilities, many changes will be made during the development time line. Changes made during development will not undergo a rigid change control system as in commercial manufacturing, but will need to be documented, justified, reviewed, and approved before use in clinical trials. A description of these changes, and their justification, will need to be discussed in the development history report. For further discussion, see Sections II.B.4 and II.B.7 of this chapter.

3. Chemistry Manufacturing and Control

Because the FDA Office of Compliance (i.e., those who are conducting the PAI) often did not have a copy of the submission that described the manufacturing process, an extra copy of the Chemistry, Manufacturing and Control (CM&C) section of the application is now required to be filed with the agency. It is also helpful to keep an extra copy available for the PAI. This extra copy has become known as the "third copy." The third copy requirement states that, for each batch of the drug product used to conduct a pivotal bioavailability or bioequivalence study or used to conduct a primary stability study, the following data should be documented and submitted:

1. The batch production record
2. The specifications and test procedures for each component and for the drug product
3. The names and addresses of the sources of the active and noncompendial inactive components and of the container closure system for the drug product
4. Results of any test performed on the components used in the manufacture of the drug product and on the drug product
5. The name and address of each contract facility involved in the manufacture, processing, packaging, or testing of the drug product and identification of the operation performed by each contract facility
6. The proposed or actual master production record, including a description of the equipment to be used for the manufacture of a commercial lot of the drug product or a comparably detailed description of the production process for a representative batch of the drug product must be provided for all initial NDAs; ANDAs must contain a proposed or actual master production record

These requirements also apply to supplements, except that the information required in the supplement is limited to that needed to support the change being submitted.

4. Development History Report

The development history report is a critical document for facilitating the PAI. This document is a historical summary of the science and rationale of the development of the API, the new drug product, and/or a history of the changes made in analytical methods during the development process. This document should be written to address all three topics—API, new drug product, or analytical methods—or it may be separated into three different reports, one report for each topic.

Regulatory agencies expect that a manufacturing process submitted in an application will yield a commercial product that is equivalent to the drug substance or clinical trial batch on which bioavailability studies, bioequivalency studies, and stability studies are conducted. This is especially critical to the clinical trial batches that were manufactured for phase III clinical trials.

To establish the link between the process used to manufacture clinical trial batches and the commercial process, the development and scale-up of the process must be appropriately documented. The logic and data that correlate production batches with clinical batches may reside in various technical reports, summary documents, or laboratory notebooks. The development history report should pull all of this information together, thus providing a summary of this information from these various sources and reference these documents where it is appropriate.

The importance of the development history report was first communicated in the FDA *Compliance Program Guidance Manual 7368.001, Pre-Approval Inspection of New Animal Drug Applications (NADA) and Abbreviated New Animal Drug Applications (ANADA)* in October 1991 [4]. In this guidance manual, the FDA inspection team is guided to inspect the data that link the manufacture and control of small scale clinical trial batches to the manufacture and control of the proposed commercial batch. This guidance manual identifies the documentation of such data in development notebooks, batch records, inventory records, and/or receiving records.

The manual then states that generally, manufacturers prepare reports that outline the experiments and data generated to develop the manufacturing process and select and identify the source and purity of the drug substance. This report should support the manufacturing process.

Although the agency referred to this summary report in their guidance manual, the development history report is not a required document under the cGMPs. As such, the absence of this report should not be listed as a deficiency in the inspection form [5].

Regardless of the absence of a legal requirement to write a development history report, it remains critical to do so for three reasons: (1) the FDA encourages the writing of it because it facilitates the PAI; (2) the document may be useful as an executive summary for the technology transfer of the process from development to production; and (3) it aids in the review of all of the work performed during the development process, ensuring that the corporation is comfortable and ready for the PAI before the submission.

There are many different issues that may be discussed in the development history report. The decision to cover a particular topic in the report is usually related to the specific nature of the development activity (e.g., manufacturing and testing issues related to fermentation production, synthetic chemical production, small molecule synthesis, biomolecule isolation, purification, etc.), and the specific type of formulation (e.g., dry product, oral liquid, parenteral, transdermal patch, etc.). When preparing the development history report, the following topics should be considered:

1. *Introduction*: a brief summary of the purpose, scope, and period covered in the document
2. *Description of the drug product*: a discussion of the history of each dosage form from the development through the formulation and process being submitted in the NDA/ANDA; for parenteral dosage forms, additional consideration to address are: extrusion force, particulate levels, metal/light sensitivity, filter compatibility and integrity, oxygen sensitivity, container requirements, preservative effectiveness, heat sensitivity, sterility test results, media fill results, list of all organisms isolated and source, etc.
3. Structure and related information regarding the drug substance
4. *Physiochemical characterization of the drug substance*: a discussion of the purity profile and in-process related substances, particle size, solubility, bulk density, polymorphism, hygroscopicity, etc.
5 *Pharmaceutical development*: a description, rationale, and history for the API and formula development of each dosage form, including a discussion of changes made and rationale for those changes made during development, a comparison of equipment used in small-scale production to equipment used in large-scale production, critical process parameters identified and how they will be controlled, granulation studies, dissolution profile, etc.
6. *Equivalence of lots manufactured at various development stages*: a discussion of equivalence of assay results (e.g., potency, related substances, etc.) or of clinical response indicators (e.g., pharmacokinetic data) for lots used in clinical trials, for lots manufactured at different scales and in different equipment or for different dosage forms
7. *Analytical development*: a chronological listing of API and drug dosage assay results and method version used, finished product testing of content uniformity, potency, friability, etc.
8. *Cleaning validation*: a discussion of rationale and data to support the cleaning validation
9. *Stability*: a summary of stability data for each dosage and package form. The data must substantiate any required or specified expiration date for the product, including any reconstituted dosage forms
10. *Specifications:* justifications of specifications for both API and drug product

11. *Conclusion*: a discussion that materials manufactured, tested, and studied in clinical trials are equivalent to materials manufactured at large scale for commercial distribution
12. *Review and approval*: by Process Development, Product Development, Quality Control/Quality Assurance, Manufacturing Operations

Although the list of possible topics to be discussed in the development history report may appear formidable, each new drug product may not include every topic listed, each topic should be discussed without too much detail, and the report should be easy to read. The details and data supporting the detail should be referenced to the original technical report and laboratory notebook.

5. Deviation Records

A deviation is any departure from an established quality standard. For development batches, these standards will be broader than those for commercial products; however, standards need to exist in the product development laboratories and should be followed. Such standards may be in the form of a standard operating procedure, a manufacturing or development batch record, a packaging order, a raw material or product specification, an analytical control procedure, a utility monitoring procedure, an equipment maintenance schedule, or any unusual occurrence. A deviation may be anticipated or unanticipated departures from the established standard and has the potential to affect the identity, strength, quality, or purity of the product.

Deviation records are reports that describes the deviation and the resulting investigation, rationale for the disposition of the deviation, follow-up actions if required, and identification of those approving the actions taken. In the development process, the deviation reporting procedure may be different from the procedure of a commercial product. Even so, all deviations must be appropriately documented, investigated, and resolved before any batch, whether for clinical trial or commercial use, may be approved.

A deviation log is helpful in summarizing deviations and their handling during a PAI. These logs allow the inspection team to quickly identify areas where departures from quality standards have occurred and allows the corporation to demonstrate that a proper action response has been made and that the system is under control. The logs are also helpful for the corporation to identify areas that may need extra attention during periodic reviews or internal quality audits.

6. Installation Qualification/Operational Qualification

Installation qualification (IQ) is the documentation of evidence that key aspects of any purchased item or installation of that item conforms to approved, written specifications. Operational qualification (OQ) is the next step in the process. OQ documents the evidence that an installed system performs as intended throughout all of the anticipated operating ranges. Examples of development equipment that should have IQ/OQ documentation available are: analytical laboratory equipment such as high-pressure liquid chromatography (HPLC) systems, dissolution equipment, and manufacturing equipment such as mills, freeze dryers, tablet presses, and chemical reactors.

This system allows one to demonstrate that equipment or systems that may affect the identity, strength, quality, or purity of the clinical trial material or new drug product are under control and perform as intended.

7. Major Changes

A change is a planned, permanent alteration or replacement of an established standard. This standard may be an analytical method, a formula, a piece of equipment, or a facility. During the PAI, the inspection team is required to evaluate all changes that may affect the new product under consideration. The inspection team is to also consider how the new product may affect other products already approved for production in the same area.

Change control, described in Section II.B.2, is the system through which changes are reviewed, justified, documented, approved, and implemented in conformance with regulatory requirements. A log trial lists all changes that are approved is helpful during the PAI. This gives the inspection team another indication of the level of control of the quality system that governs the manufacture of the new product.

Change control is a system of commercial production. However, change is an integral part of the development process. The changes that occur in development need to be made quickly and often. As a result, a system of "change documentation" may be more appropriate than a "change control" system. It is critical that changes made during the development time line are documented and justified. These changes should be reviewed before the batch is approved to ensure that the process remains within the application, usually the IND, commitments. These change documents and reports of change review will need to be available for the PAI. These documents will most likely be a part of the batch disposition record.

8. Organizational Chart

Organizational charts are helpful tools that demonstrate three items that are important for the FDA inspection team to establish: (1) that an adequate number of personnel are available to perform and supervise the manufacture, processing, packaging, or holding of a drug product (21 CFR 211.25); (2) that a proper chain of responsibility has been established in supervisors of manufacturing processes;

and (3) that there is appropriate separation of responsibilities for manufacturing operations and the quality unit.

These charts will need to be available from both the development organizations and the commercial manufacturing organizations.

9. Products List

As was discussed in Section II.B.7, the inspection team is required to evaluate how the new product may affect other products already approved for production in the same area. Having a list of materials that are already approved for production facilitates this portion of the inspection. An inspection team member may quickly assess what potential may exist for cross-contamination in the production area.

10. Site Plan Drawings

Site plan drawings are helpful to the successful completion of the PAI. These drawings quickly show how the facility is constructed and controlled, and include the following:

1. *Floor plan*: demonstrates proper segregation of areas by walls, air locks, and doors; these plans are useful to demonstrate people and equipment flow, showing that clean personnel and equipment do not cross paths with dirty personnel and equipment
2. *Facility and grounds*: these drawings show the relationship of all of the buildings and facilities to each other; they may demonstrate proper separation of products that are manufactured in different buildings and proper security of the general facility

These drawings should be available for facilities used in clinical trial material production as well as those where commercial products will be produced.

11. Stability Data

It is the FDA field investigator's responsibility to determine the validity of the data that support the product stability. The inspection team is directed to conduct an audit of the data that were furnished in the application. Therefore, data from all stability indicating analyses should be readily available, as well as the stability protocol. The stability indicating analyses will differ from product to product. It is during the development process that stability conditions and testing methods are defined. Some examples of stability data that should be made available for the PAI are: HPLC raw data from potency and related substance testing, and moisture content tests.

This can be an enormous amount of data. Data management is an important issue for the PAI and is covered in Section III. Chapter 4 includes further discussion of stability data management.

12. Standard Operating Procedures

Standard operating procedures (SOPs) are a set of written instructions that set policy or describe an operation for a designated operational area. A set of SOPs that are relevant to the manufacture, processing, packaging, or testing of the clinical trial materials and the commercial drug product should be made available during the inspection. It is usually helpful to have a copy of the SOP index so that the inspection team may quickly see which SOPs may be requested during the PAI.

13. Training Records

It is a cGMP requirement (21 CFR 211.25 a,b) that personnel have education, training, or experience that enables them to perform their assigned task. Training records should be available to the inspection team during the PAI. This enables the team to evaluate that appropriate training was conducted. These training records should include the training curriculum for each individual, as well as the list of completed courses. These records should be made available for all personnel who manufacture, process, package, test, or release clinical trial materials and the commercial product.

14. Utility Drawings

Utility drawings are essential to the successful completion of the PAI. These drawings quickly show how the utilities are constructed and controlled, and include:

1. *Heating, Ventilation, and Air Conditioning (HVAC)*: HVAC drawings are helpful in demonstrating that there is no cross-contamination issue regarding airflow between manufacturing areas (pilot plants and commercial plants). It is helpful to have schematic drawings of the floor plan that indicate pressure differentials between rooms, common hallways, and air interlocks.
2. *Water*: Water system drawings are important to show that the water system is properly constructed with no dead-legs in the system. It is helpful to indicate the testing points with a cross-reference to the water testing plan.

As with other documents already discussed, the drawings that need to be available during the PAI pertain to both clinical trial manufacturing facilities and commercial manufacturing facilities.

15. Validation Records

The concept of validation relates to the documented evidence that a system does what it purports to do. A written plan, or protocol, is a document that defines how validation will be conducted. The protocol may include test parameters, product characteristics, production equipment specifications and settings, and decision points on what constitutes acceptable test results. Three types of validation protocols should be available during the PAI: cleaning, manufacturing process, and analytical methods. Any data associated with a completed protocol should also be made available.

C. How Documents Will Be Reviewed

Different inspection teams have different inspection styles. As a result, there may not be any two PAIs that are conducted exactly the same way. In fact, it would be surprising if any two inspections were the same. Some inspection teams may desire to review the documents in a conference room where there is plenty of room to spread the documents on tables to compare them more easily. Other inspection teams will want to review documentation in the laboratories and manufacturing areas. There will often be a combination of the two methods

In general, the role of inspection team in conducting a PAI is to assure cGMP compliance, verify the accuracy and authenticity of the data that are contained in the application, and report any other observations that may impact the firm's ability to manufacture the product in compliance with cGMPs. Listed below are FDA expectations and a discussion of how documents will be reviewed during the PAI.

In conducting the PAI the FDA expects to ensure that firms:

1. *Have demonstrated bioequivalency between clinical trial batches and production and scale batches*: This is done by comparing the documentation of the manufacturing process used for manufacturing clinical trial batches to the documentation of the manufacturing process used for producing the commercial product. This is usually performed by examining pivotal clinical trial batch records, especially for the clinical trial materials that were manufactured and used in phase III clinical trials. Pivotal clinical trial batches include stability, bioavailability, and bioequivalency batches, and are compared to scale-up and validation batches at the commercial facility. This review also includes raw analytical data that bridge the pivotal clinical trial batches to the commercial batches. A summary discussion of the above should be contained in the development history report.

2. *Are in compliance with the cGMPs*: This is done by examining equipment maintenance records, SOPs for proper review and approval, and for

deviation reports and change control reports for the same. IQ/OQ documents are reviewed as well as training records. The focus of the FDA is usually on the commercial facility; however, this review could go back into clinical trial manufacturing facilities. Several companies have experienced the PAI reaching back into development activities, especially in the analytical development laboratories.

3. *Have submitted factual data*: This is done by a side-by-side comparison of data that are submitted in the application with raw analytical data. The inspection team may ask to see the raw data for a particular HPLC tracing and compare it to a HPLC tracing that is contained in the application. It is also done by comparing the manufacturing process contained in the application with the manufacturing process contained in batch records.

4. *Have the ability to manufacture the product in accordance with their registration submissions*: This is done by a comparison of the manufacturing description submitted in the application to original development batch records. This also includes a cGMP compliance assessment at the commercial manufacturing site as well as a review of the various validation protocols and associated data.

5. *Assure the accuracy of their analytical methods*: A review of laboratory methods will be performed to determine compliance with the method as well as proper review and approval of the method. Included in this methodology review will be an examination of the methods transfer documents that ensure that methods run in a development laboratory will give the same results as methods run in a production control laboratory.

III. PREPARING DOCUMENTS FOR THE PAI

Now that one knows what documents need to be available for the PAI, the task is to manage the large numbers of documents. This task is confounded by the fact that many pharmaceutical companies are multinational, international, or transnational corporations. This means that clinical trial material manufacturing and development work may have been conducted in the United States, whereas the commercial API may come from Europe and the commercial drug product may be sourced from Puerto Rico.

It has been said of the PAI that there is a "100% preparation for a 10% inspection." One never knows which document will be requested for review during the PAI. Therefore, all documents need to be readied and made available, with the understanding that the inspection team will not review everything that is prepared. This can be very frustrating to individuals who have devoted their time and efforts to write and prepare the documentation, only to have it "ignored" during the PAI. There may be a corollary to Murphy's law, which reads: the one document that is not available will be the one that the FDA requests.

A. Assign Responsibility

The first step in managing the vast numbers of PAI documents is to assign responsibility to those who will write, review, approve, and protect all documents, both development and commercial manufacturing documents. Protection of the documents is defined as the storage of the documents and distribution of the documents in preparation for the PAI, or distribution of the documents when they are requested during the PAI.

WRAP (W = written; R = reviewed; A = approved; P = protected) may serve as a convenient acronym to remind the PAI readiness team of the documents and process that are required to "wrap-up" a successful PAI.

The assignment of responsibility for various documents will vary according to the size and organization of individual corporations. A PAI Documents Responsibility matrix may be designed (Figure 1) that identifies what documents will be available and what individual will be responsible for writing, reviewing, approving, and protecting the various documents. An individual such as project manager may be responsible for designing the matrix and seeing that the

	Doc.	Analyt Devel.	API Devel	Form Devel.	Manuf. Site	Plant Engr.	QA	QC	Reg. Affairs	Site QC Labs	Stabil. Labs	Tech. Serv.
						Job Group						
1	Batch Record		W	W	W,R		R	R,A,P				
2	Change Control		W	W	W,R		R	R,A,P				W
3	CM&C						R		W,P			
4	Devel. History	W	W	W	R		R	R,A,P		R		R
5	Deviation Report	W	W	W	W,R		R	R,A,P		W,R		W
6	IQ/OQ				R		R	R,A,P				W
7	Changes	W	W	W	W,R		R	R,A,P	R	W,R		W
8	Org. Chart				W,P		R					
9	Prod. List				W,P		R					
10	Site Plans				W,P		R					
11	Stability Data	W,R					R	R,A			W,R,P	
12	SOPs	W	W	W	W		R	R,A,P		W	W	
13	Training Records	W	W	W	W		R	P		W	W	
14	Utility Drawings					W,R,P	R					
15	Valid. Records						R	R,A				W,R,P

Figure 1 Responsibility for PAI documents. (W, write; R, review; A, approve; P, protect (store and distribute).

documents are made available, on schedule, before the PAI. The following is an example of the distribution of responsibilities for various PAI documents.

1. Analytical Development

The analytical development chemist is responsible for developing analytical methodologies for testing the API, excipients, and the new drug product. These analytical methods will change over the years of conducting clinical trials. The analytical chemist is responsible for writing the history report that describes all of the various methodologies that have been developed. This report lists all of the methods used to release clinical trial materials for use under the IND, and a justification for changes that were made in the method. It is a type of method genealogy that demonstrates that clinical trial materials were under cGMP control at the time of use, regardless of the age of the data.

A second major document that is the responsibility of the analytical development chemist is the methods transfer documentation. When the servicing laboratory through development is different than the one that will routinely conduct the assays during manufacturing, the methods transfer will provide assurance that the transferred assays will be conducted in the same manner, with the same results.

The methods transfer may include methods used in the API, dosage form assays, assays for excipients, in-process assays, and assays for stability. This transfer document may also address analytical methods used in the cleaning validation, ruggedness testing, equipment maintenance systems and records, and the validation protocol for methods transfer including the protocol and results. The qualification of analytical equipment, current control laboratory procedures, and current specifications may also be addressed.

Other documents for which the analytical chemist is responsible is the documentation of deviations that have occurred during the release of clinical trial materials, SOPs as they apply to the analytical development division, and training records for their staff.

Depending on the size of the corporation and organizational staffing, the analytical development chemist may also be the one responsible for the collection and review of stability data.

2. API Development

The process development scientist is responsible for developing the synthetic route for manufacturing the active ingredient, frequently called the bulk drug substance. In this role, they will write manufacturing instructions that will become a part of the batch record. Also included in this batch record will be documents that record and justify changes made to each manufacturing instruction, changes that were made to the development equipment, documentation of any deviations that occurred, and SOPs and related training as they apply to the role of the Development Scientist.

One of the major documents prepared by the development scientist is the development history report. This report was discussed in section II.B.4. This report is not submitted with the NDA/ANDA, but should be written and available at the time of submission.

3. Formulation Development

The formulation development scientist is responsible for developing the process of formulating the new drug product. The role of the formulation development scientist parallels the role of the API development scientist and is responsible for the same document types as they apply to the product formulation organization.

4. Manufacturing Site

The manufacturing site (production) personnel are responsible for several documents as they relate to transferring the process to the respective commercial production site, and the validation of the process at the site. Development personnel are responsible for the documents that apply to the manufacturing sites for clinical trial materials. These documents include batch records, change control records, deviation reports, IQ/OQ documents as they relate to the specific equipment being used in the process, a list of major changes in the facility, organization charts, a list of current products being manufactured at the facility, site plans, and SOPs and related training records.

It is important that the commercial production personnel review the development history report that relates to the process that has been transferred to the commercial facility. The review of this document is important because it facilitates the technology transfer process. The development history report will identify potential manufacturing problems and how they are to be controlled.

5. Plant Engineering

Plant Engineering is responsible for generating and maintaining current plans and drawings for manufacturing utilities used in both clinical trial facilities and commercial manufacturing facilities. These utilities consist of, at minimum, HVAC, water, and floor plan drawings. It is also this area that will most likely control the documentation for building, utility, instrumentation, and equipment maintenance.

6. Quality Assurance

Quality Assurance (QA) is the division that facilitates the establishment of corporate quality policy. In addition, the QA division will host the FDA inspection team during the PAI. The various documentation for PAIs—e.g., manufacturing records, development history reports, and laboratory raw data—do not belong to the QA unit. They are, however, responsible for auditing and review of the documents that are discussed further in Section III.B.

7. Quality Control

The Quality Control (QC) unit's responsibilities are defined in 21 CFR 211.22. As such, QC is responsible for PAI documents such as the batch records of lots manufactured for clinical trials, as well as the batch records of the validation lots at the commercial facility. These batch records contain the items listed in Section II.B.1 and include change control records and deviation records.

QC is responsible for reviewing and approving the various development history reports (i.e., analytical, API, drug product). They are also responsible for the control and approval of IQ/OQ documents, and the review and approval of stability data and validation records. These validation records include the process validation protocol, equipment validation protocol, and the cleaning validation protocol.

Included in QC's responsibilities is the approval of SOPs used in GMP operations. QC may also be responsible for their associated training records.

8. Regulatory Affairs

The Regulatory Affairs representative is responsible for collating all of the submission information into one coherent submission document. They are also responsible for submission documents throughout the development process, which includes INDs and related supplements, NDA/ANDA amendments, and annual reports.

Regulatory Affairs is also responsible for all minutes of presubmission FDA meetings, and other key correspondence with the FDA. The Regulatory Affairs representative may also play a role in reviewing changes to the facility or process that may result in a supplement, amendment, or annual report. Preparing these documents for the PAI is discussed in Sections III.B, C, and D.

9. Site QC Laboratories

The QC laboratories at the commercial site are responsible for the same types of documents as the analytical development chemist is for the development methodology. The site QC personnel are responsible for conducting the method transfer and method validation at the commercial control laboratories.

10. Stability Laboratories

Some corporations have identified a separate group that conducts stability studies and that is responsible for the generation, review, and approval of all stability data. This group would be responsible for quick retrieval of all stability data during the PAI. They may also be requested to produce SOPs and associated training documents as they relate to the stability area responsibilities.

11. Technical Services

The Technical Services personnel are generally associated with a commercial facility. They are responsible for the validation of the manufacturing process and evaluation of proposed changes to the process, and they assist in deviation investigations and conduct IQ/OQ activities for facilities, utilities, and equipment. As such, the Technical Service personnel should be responsible for the corresponding documentation.

It is also critical that the Technical Services personnel review the development history report to improve the odds of a seamless process transfer from development to commercial manufacturing.

B. Process for Reviewing Documents

As the development of a new pharmaceutical product progresses, many changes will occur. Changes will be made in the synthetic steps of manufacturing the API. Changes will be made in the analytical methods that are used to test the API, as well as the formulated drug product and excipients. Changes will be made in the formulation during the development process.

These formulation changes will likely be not only minor changes in ingredients of a set formulation, but major changes in the formulation eventually chosen to be marketed. It may be that the formulation changes from an oral liquid to a capsule, then to a tablet, then on to some other formulation. These changes will have occurred over several years.

It has been clear that the commercial lots be manufactured under cGMPs and have associated documentation for proof. It has also been shown that clinical trial materials must be made under cGMPs. This implies that all data must be readily available, reviewable, generated, and reported with integrity. Although, to date, the agency has focused on bridging phase III clinical trial materials to the commercial process, it would be prudent to document that all clinical trial materials were compliant with the cGMPs, regardless of the phase of development or the age of the data.

It is critical that all of the documents listed in Section II.B be reviewed. These documents must be reviewed for accuracy, integrity, and ease of retrieval. This review is usually accomplished by a QA internal audit of the submission.

QA conducts the audit in cooperation with individuals in Analytical Development, Process Development, Pharmaceutical Development, Manufacturing personnel, Engineering, Quality Control, Regulatory Affairs, Technical Service personnel, and others.

One method of conducting the audit is to simulate the PAI process. The FDA inspection team will have a copy of the CM&C section of the application and will determine if factual data have been submitted to the agency. The FDA will do this by asking to review the raw data that are submitted in the various sections of the applications. They will review manufacturing instructions and batch records and compare them to the process description in the application. The team will compare excipients and raw materials used, and they will check equipment used and compare them to the process description. The FDA will request raw analytical data from release tests of the batches that are reviewed and from stability studies that justify the expiry date of the new drug product. During the inspection, a review of the development history report(s) will be performed, which identifies critical process control parameters and determines if the parameters have, indeed, been controlled in the commercial process. They will review the validation documents for process, analytical methods, and cleaning validation.

There will be a review of the documents that demonstrate that the manufacturing facilities are under cGMP control. The FDA will review water monitoring data as well as the drawings of the facility, utility diagrams, and maintenance program documents. They will review SOPs that control the production areas of clinical trial manufacturing and commercial production. Also, a review of the analytical methodology for validated methods will be conducted to determine if the analytical methods have been properly transferred.

In a like manner, the QA audit should review each of the documents listed in Section II.B, starting with the CM&C section of the application, and duplicate the above process. This review should be conducted as early as possible before the application is submitted to correct any errors in the submission document. Error corrections are discussed in Section III.C.

The review should focus first on the documentation related to the definitive stability, biobatch, scale-up, and validation batches. From that point, the next review should focus on pivotal clinical trial batches. The pivotal clinical trials batches would include any of the above batches as well as batches that were used in bioavailability or bioequivalency studies. These may be the API batches that demonstrate the equivalency of two different synthetic routes, or they may be the formulation batches that demonstrate the equivalency between a capsule formulation and a tablet formulation.

The review should consider other clinical trial batches. Generally, a genealogy of clinical trial batches is included in the application, and the FDA may review any batch listed. This review should compare clinical trial batches to the IND in force at the time of manufacture.

In each of these reviews, one should examine the raw analytical data. It is not sufficient to review progress reports or summary reports. The review should reach all of the way back to original laboratory notebooks.

C. Correct Problems

As one conducts the review of the current definitive stability, biobatch, scale-up, and validation batches, it is unlikely that gross errors will be detected. However, as one reviews the clinical trial documents that were generated years ago, the probability for finding errors will greatly increase. This is due, in part, to the dynamic nature of the cGMPs. The documentation practices that may be considered "current" today may be different from the practices several years ago when the development process and clinical trials began.

The development history report is another tool used to detect issues in development design. The writing and review of the development history report affords the opportunity to reflect on the entire development process. It provides a broad perspective on the design logic of experiments and clinical trials conducted. During the review of the development history report, "holes" may be detected. These holes may be the absence of raw data that demonstrate particle size equivalency in milling processes, or it may be the discovery of a critical process parameter that remains elusive to control.

Writing and reviewing the development history report may identify gaps in the development process, but it will not repair the gap. To repair the gap, additional data may be required to be collected. For example, in the illustration above where particle size data was inadvertently not collected, it may become necessary to collect the data. This may be performed by accessing a small amount of material from the reserve samples that are required by 21 CFR 211.170. If this is not possible, perhaps there is other evidence that demonstrates that particle size is not a critical parameter that needs to be controlled.

During the review of the batch records and associated documents (i.e., deviation reports, change control documents, and analytical data), if a discrepancy or incomplete data are found, the number one rule to follow is: under no circumstances should any document in the original batch record be modified.

If a discrepancy or error is found, an addendum to the batch record may be added. In this addendum, comments may be added to clarify, and deviation reports may be added to justify. In the deviation report, issues with changes, accountability, or assay results should be evaluated. In general, the "batch worthiness" is being justified. For example, in the review of a batch record, if it is found that an operator had unintentionally not signed the record for addition of a raw material, instead of filling in the missing initials, QC should write a deviation report describing the error and the investigation that compared the quality attributes of the final product to the specifications. The conclusion may be drawn that the raw material was added, regardless of the lack of operator initials, because the reaction went to completion, or the final product met specifications.

If several discrepancies of a similar nature are found, it would be prudent to prepare an addendum that explains the improvement in the quality system which controls the particular process being reviewed.

In the event that an original document cannot be located, the batch history may be reconstructed, but the reconstruction must be from raw data, not from opinions or conclusions found in other reports. For example, if the documentation for content uniformity of a clinical trial batch cannot be located, the data may be collected from reserve samples or a rerun of that clinical trial manufacturing process. The action taken will depend on the criticality of the data needed.

If a discrepancy is found, during the review of compliance to regulatory commitments, it is important that it be resolved through appropriate action with the agency. This may entail the submission of an amendment or supplement, or the issue may be resolved in the next annual report.

Depending on the way the issue is resolved, a delay in the submission may be inevitable. Due to the cost of development and the lost opportunities in the market place, a delay of submission will be at high cost to the corporation. A delay may also be at high cost to the patient who is waiting for treatment.

If a discrepancy is found in the writing or review of the analytical development history report, additional data must be collected. For example, if the justification for a method change was not based on raw data comparing the two methods, method equivalency can be demonstrated by collecting further data. This data could be gathered on the original batches if sufficient materials are available through the reserve sample, or may be collected on equivalent batches where sufficient materials are available. Similar data can be collected to demonstrate formulation mixture and USP method compatibility if it had not been previously demonstrated.

Whatever corrective action is taken, it must be documented so that the integrity of the original document is never questioned by the FDA during the PAI.

D. Decide on a Location for PAI Documents

In an age in which the PAI for one drug product may be conducted at several different sites and on several continents, the management of the document location becomes critical. Various corporations have responded to this situation in several different ways. Some companies will gather all of the relevant documents in one location where they will be available for the inspection. These documents, for some companies, will be the original documents; other companies will provide a photocopy of the original. If photocopies are used, some companies require the use of a stamp that indicates that the photocopy is an exact duplicate of the original document, and is accompanied by the initials and date of the person making the copy.

Other companies have retained the original document at the site which "owns" the document. When information is requested from that particular document, a facsimile (fax) is transmitted via the telephone system. This practice has worked for some companies, but it must be recognized that the success of the PAI may depend on the reliability of the fax operator, fax equipment, or telephone lines between sites.

Another strategy is similar to the one above. The original document is retained at the site of "ownership." When the document is requested, a company employee will hand carry the original document to the inspection site. With international inspections, this strategy can be costly and frustrating for the inspection team waiting for the document to arrive.

The recommended strategy represents a unique blend of the above practices. It facilitates the PAI to have all of the documents at the site of inspection when the inspection team arrives. However, it is always a risk to allow an original document to leave the controlled environment of its ""owner." Therefore, it is recommended that photocopies of the original documents be available at the inspection sites, with the offer to the inspection team, that if an original document is necessary, a review of its photocopy can proceed while the original is being transported to the inspection site. This avoids delay in the review and demonstrates a willingness to provide the needed documentation.

A level of uncertainty exists concerning the location of the PAI. For example, the API will be manufactured at a different site from that of the drug product. The API and drug product may be tested in laboratories located at sites different from where the materials were manufactured. Stability studies may be conducted at laboratories that are different from the laboratories conducting the release assays. Finally, the product may be packaged, stored, and distributed at different sites.

It is important to communicate with the district FDA office and the local FDA office during the development process and, especially, at the time of technology transfer from development to the commercial facility. Contact should be made early to determine, if possible, where the agency will need the documents for the inspection. This will minimize unnecessary work and delays.

It must also be recognized that the photocopying of all related documents is time-consuming and expensive. However, it will be more costly to not photocopy the required documents and delay the approval of the new drug product. As was previously stated, some PAI preparation activities will never be reviewed by the inspection team. Understanding this concept avoids frustration later.

IV. PROSPECTIVE DOCUMENTATION VERSUS RETROSPECTIVE DOCUMENTATION

The review and correction of documents that were created in the past has been described as "retrospective documentation." The concept of retrospective documentation provides a tool for demonstrating that all clinical trial materials complied with cGMP during the entire multiyear process of development. Retrospective documentation is the process of reconstructing the history of the development of a new pharmaceutical product. Unlike the reconstruction of an historical event that may be based on providing a plausible story, retrospective documentation may not be based on opinion. It must be based on scientific evidence and raw data that are collected and reported accurately.

The retrospective review of all documents that affect the outcome of a PAI is necessary during a period of rapid change. It must be performed under the highest integrity. However, retrospective documentation is time-consuming and tedious. There may be difficulty in locating all of the pertinent data, which will require collection of additional data.

The current paradigm for preparing a PAI is to treat the PAI as an event. The preparation for the PAI must become a process (i.e., it must become prospective and a part of the drug development process). This process requires the creation of a quality system that controls the writing, reviewing, approval, and protection of documents throughout the entire development process. For example, the development history report must be written on a continuous basis as interim reports. These reports may be detailed technical reports that can easily be summarized for a brief development history summary with references to the detailed reports, should the inspection team wish to review the detail.

The prospective process requires a management system for distributing documents to the inspection site at the appropriate time. It requires a system for better scheduling the inspection so that documents may be sent to the proper inspection site.

V. RESULTS OF A FAILURE TO DOCUMENT

Failure to document properly or appropriately may lead to several different results:

1. *Delay in approval*: resulting in lost opportunity costs to the corporation and delay in effective treatment to patients
2. *Withhold approval*: resulting in the same as a delay in approval except more costly to both the corporation and the patient; the consequences of failing a PAI are discussed in Chapter 6
3. *Loss of trust*: between the corporation and the FDA
4. *It is poor science*: this is self-explanatory
5. *Integrity violation*: as discussed in Section II.A.1, this could result in a regulatory "hold" on all of the company's applications; in the early 1990s, the industry saw the Application Integrity Policy enforced
6. *Market recalls*: which result in lost revenue, and market and patient confidence
7. *Legal violations*: resulting in costly fines and imprisonment

VI. CONCLUSIONS

The adage, "There is only one opportunity to make a good first impression," is applicable to the PAI. The PAI is a "picture" taken at a point in time by the FDA that confirms or disproves the firm's ability to manufacture a new drug product in compliance with all of the application requirements.

Proper documentation is the key to making a good first impression. Without proper and adequate documentation, it will be impossible to demonstrate a properly developed pharmaceutical product. Without good documentation there will be delays in approving the new product, increased costs, delays in getting new drugs to patients in need; it calls into question all the work that the firm has performed, and it appears to be poor science.

REFERENCES

1. J. A. DiMase, R. W. Hansen, H. G. Grabowski, L. Lasagna, The cost of innovation in the pharmaceutical industry, *J. Health Economics* 10:2 (1991).
2. Food and Drug Administration Commissioner's Exchange Meeting, Proceedings, Itasca, Illinois, 1991, pp. 17–18.
3. FDA, *Food and Drug Administration Compliance Program Guidance Manual 7346.832, Pre-Approval inspections/investigations*, 1994, p. 5.

4. FDA, *Food and Drug Administration Compliance Program Guidance Manual 7368.001, Pre-Approved Inspection of New Animal Drug Applications (NADA) and Abbreviated New Animal Drug Applications (ANADA)*, 1991.
5. W. Paulson, ed., Development reports should discuss formulation evaluations, *The Gold Sheet* 26:6 (1992).

9

Technology Transfer and Scale-Up

Elizabeth MacLennan Troll
Guilford Pharmaceuticals, Inc., Baltimore, Maryland

I. INTRODUCTION

The goal of technology transfer and scale-up is to show, through process control, that any modifications made from conception to implementation have been appropriately evaluated and documented, and that the product is safe, pure, and effective. The Food and Drug Administration (FDA) pre-approval and post-approval inspections focus on the review of data generated from the development plan used to define the manufacture and evaluation of the proposed drug product or device. The overall development plan should include a standardized vehicle for evaluating the technology transfer and scale-up process.

The vehicle should take into account the transfer considerations between the five key elements of the change control process (Figure 1). The technology transfer points are represented by the arrows in the figure. A sample vehicle that could be utilized would be a series of reports issued at each transfer point and audited (before issuance) for 100% data integrity.

Each report would contain a summary of factual data, supplemented with scientific judgment defining the meaning of the data, and a set of conclusions or recommendations for process controls based on the facts. The overall collection of the completed and approved reports would represent the documentation trail of the technology transfer process.

The advantage to an "audit-as-you-go" program is the ability to identify and correct documentation issues as they occur. This is a proactive approach.

215

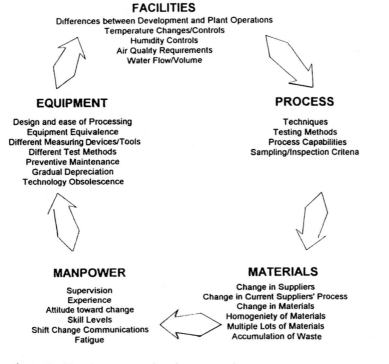

FACILITIES
Differences between Development and Plant Operations
Temperature Changes/Controls
Humidity Controls
Air Quality Requirements
Water Flow/Volume

EQUIPMENT

Design and ease of Processing
Equipment Equivalence
Different Measuring Devices/Tools
Different Test Methods
Preventive Maintenance
Gradual Depreciation
Technology Obsolescence

PROCESS

Techniques
Testing Methods
Process Capabilities
Sampling/Inspection Criteria

MANPOWER

Supervision
Experience
Attitude toward change
Skill Levels
Shift Change Communications
Fatigue

MATERIALS

Change in Suppliers
Change in Current Suppliers' Process
Change in Materials
Homogeniety of Materials
Multiple Lots of Materials
Accumulation of Waste

Figure 1   The change control cycle.

Evaluating the document trail at the end of the development process is a formidable task. The volume of data that accumulates over the years of development will cause the review effort to take on herculean proportions. Changes in project personnel, corporate leadership/ownership, material traceability, equipment modification/identification, site-to-site transfers, etc., compound the difficulty of the task.

A well-organized plan of review that anticipates and documents these types of changes is an invaluable tool in preserving the audit trail of the technology transfer process. It can prevent a reviewer from having unexpected audit observations that could cast doubt on the safety, purity, and efficacy of the product/process.

II. THE TECHNOLOGY TRANSFER MASTER PLAN

The Technology Transfer master plan can be broken into three elements that are applicable to all drug dosage forms and medical devices. The three elements can be reviewed throughout the developmental process or at certain "go/no-go" points in development. The elements can be rereviewed when the product or process is site transferred or modified. A description of the three elements follows.

A. Element 1: Documentation Practices

Primary documentation includes all original batch records, raw testing data, raw material testing records, packaging component testing records, and all developmental, validation, and clinical data reports. Support documentation includes all purchase orders, inventory records, distribution reports, and major handling systems (water, air, lighting, power, and security).

B. Element 2: Technical Writing Styles

Audiences for the written word change as the product or process matures to the eventual instructions for the manufacture of the commercially distributed product. An overall awareness of the current audience and the final audience will help technical data generators build reports that accurately convey the details of the product or process.

C. Element 3: Illustration of Equivalence

Multiple options are available to illustrate equivalence. These include but are not limited to: (1) side by side/step by step comparisons; (2) flow diagrams; (3) critical step definitions; and (4) physical space comparisons (tank, building, filing equipment, drawings).

The concepts presented herein are designed to be a guideline for developing a technology transfer master plan to fit any product or process. The elements listed are common to all products and processes. Each element is defined and accompanied by a list of issues significant to the understanding of the element.

Where practical, suggestions for issue definition are included. These suggestions can be considered tools of the technology transfer process. The tools outlined in this chapter can make the most complicated product/process easy to understand if they are used at the point of data generation.

III. TECHNOLOGY TRANSFER MASTER PLAN: ELEMENT
ONE—DOCUMENTATION PRACTICES

The credo, "If you didn't document it, you didn't do it," is especially applicable to the technology transfer and scale-up process. The document trail that begins on the bench and ends with commercial distribution is the trail an auditor uses to assure the reviewers that any modifications made to the product or process do not impact the safety, purity, or efficacy of the drug product or device.

The complexity of the overall developmental process can confuse an inexperienced auditor/reviewer. No matter how complex, all products/processes have two common documentation sections. The sections are divided into the primary batch record data and the documents that support the batch record data. It is important to understand the difference between the primary documentation and support documentation. The FDA will focus on primary documentation to evaluate the product under review for safety, purity, and efficacy. The FDA will focus on support documentation to evaluate the current Good Manufacturing Procedures (cGMP) compliance status of the facility(ies) in which the primary documentation was generated.

Documentation nomenclature and the manner in which data is recorded are additional issues worthy of review. Setting standards for the "written word" is important to assure that gathered facts are clear and understandable. Suggestions for standardization of these issues are included in Sections III.C and D.

A. Primary Documentation

Primary documentation includes all original batch records, raw testing data, raw material testing records, packaging component testing recorded, and all developmental, validation, and clinical data reports. Raw materials and packaging components are combined through a defined and documented process, and produce a finished product. The written record of these activities is generally referred to as the batch record. Developmental, validation, and clinical data reports are summaries of the activities and data generated during selected phases of product/process development. Collectively, these reports support the claims of safety, purity, and efficacy of the drug product. The FDA will review these records to evaluate the safety, purity, and efficacy of the proposed drug product.

Original data can be found in a variety of sources: bound or unbound laboratory notebooks, individual data reports, original chromatograms, data printouts from electronic equipment/recording devices, hand-reported data on individual paper pages, electronically recorded data in paperless systems. This type of data is generally "not repeatable." Two main concerns exist for this type of documentation: security and authenticity. Suggestions for the standardization of format for original data can be found in Section III.D.

B. Supporting Documentation

Supporting documentation includes all purchase orders, inventory records, and distribution reports. The significance of these records can be easily overlooked because they usually are not considered by many as part of the process. Many consider these tools used to get the building blocks of the process to the facility to turn them into the finished products. In reality, they are a basis for the FDA to be able to evaluate your product/process. The FDA is a federal agency with its basis in interstate commerce. By reviewing these types of documents, the agency can establish that you have engaged in interstate commerce by accepting and paying for materials from other states and countries. These documents can also serve as authenticity verification for potential misbranded or unapproved sources of raw materials or components. The FDA can also use these documents to verify the authenticity of the actual shipment of raw materials or components.

Another set of support records would include all of the physical data that surround the production process, including major handling systems such as water, air (heat, ventilation, and air conditioning [HVAC], compressed, clean), lighting, power, security (for controlled drugs), facility drawings, and preventative maintenance schedules. These systems have tremendous impact on how well a process is controlled. A review of these records will help an FDA inspector evaluate the effectivity of change control procedures. Effective change control procedures gives a reviewer confidence that cGMP compliance will be maintained on an on-going basis.

Each of the five key units of change control outlined in Figure 1 has an associated group of records defining acceptability criteria. The acceptability criteria may be different depending on the facility. For illustration purposes, consider the flow of deionized water into a research and development laboratory and a manufacturing facility:

> Many laboratories use an "on-demand" deionized water system for the manufacture of sample formulations. Flow rate and temperature of the water in this environment is not always monitored and recorded as part of the experiment. Bioburden levels of the water are effected by flow rate and temperature. The manufacturing facility will have a deionized water system that has flow and temperature control. The bioburden of this water system will be a key element for plant process control. If the product's bioburden requirements are not evaluated in the research and development laboratory environment, it is possible that the product cannot be produced in the manufacturing facility.

An evaluation of the process capability of the laboratory environment and the potential manufacturing site is an important piece of the technology transfer process. In our example, the flow rate and temperature of water to the manufacturing facility may not be able to meet the demands of the formulation. Using the "audit-as-you-go" concept, one would know before scale-up production that the formulation may not be able to be made in the intended facility. The financial benefit to the company is that the company will not make a batch that by definition will not meet the process criteria.

FDA reviewers and auditors alike will use this type of information when evaluating site-to-site product transfers. If sites A and B are not environmentally equivalent or do not have similar system capacities, then questions could be raised on how the differences between the two facilities can affect the safety, efficacy, and purity of the drug product. Additionally, if change control procedures are not equivalent, the FDA will have limited assurance that cGMP compliance will be met on an on-going basis.

C. Documentation Nomenclature

Each one of the two documentation sections require certain markings that associate them to the particular product/process. If one were to think of the entire body of work as a process map, these would be the legend markings. A well-planned technology transfer process will have a clear set of legends defined for the process, including part numbers, product name, equipment identifications, day and date of work performed, location of work performed, and signatures of persons performing and/or witnessing the work performed.

1. Part Numbers

A part number is an identification code attached to any item that is part of a product or process. Generally, a part number begins as an inventory designation for a raw material, component, or product. The logical section of the part number sequence may be driven by the immediate need of the moment, not by the overall need of the product/process. During the course of development, these initial part numbers may be replaced by more meaningful part numbers.

Some developmental plans call for the reallocation of materials, previously designated for research and development, for use in the product intended for commercial distribution. This change in status from research and development to GMP status may be predicated by cost and availability of the material. Some reviewers may have issues with having two different statuses applied to the same lot of material. A strong document trail that clearly defines the change in status is an essential component for supporting the release of the commercially distributed product. The master specification is a logical place to archive these types of changes. The evolution of the master specification from "For Research and Development" to "For Material Release" provides the reviewer with a complete audit trail of change.

As a reviewer moves through the body of work associated with a particular product/process, a change in numbering may be confusing. The reviewer may not understand that two different designations are meant for the same material. It may be advisable to supply the reviewer with a cross-reference to aid in the review process.

The following questions can be asked by a reviewer in an attempt to understand the level of change control being applied to the part number assignment system. Who has authority to assign part numbers? Is their a logical sequence in the assignment of these numbers? If a material/product is to be discontinued, will the part number be retired? Can a retired part number ever be reactivated? The policies and procedures used to assign part numbers should included provisions to address these issues.

2. Product Name

Product names are generally the most modified piece of documentation within the body of developmental work. Usually, the first identification code attached to a product or process is generated from a laboratory environment. It may be an idea from an inventor or a request from the Marketing Department. Someone will begin experiments and will record information related to the idea. If it is raw material, component, or product, a part number may be assigned as an inventory designation for the idea. Eventually, it will become a bonafide project and receive a project number (also a part number). As application time draws near, the "officially recognized" name may be assigned. A trade name may also be chosen at this point of the development process.

Changes in nomenclature may be confusing to a reviewer. The reviewer may not understand that different designations are meant for the same material. It is advisable to supply the reviewer with a cross-reference to aid in the review process.

3. Equipment Identifications

Equipment identifications are facility-related part numbers and can fall victim to the same issues as general part number assignments. A record of equipment identification numbers may be appropriate to assure that similar pieces of equipment do not receive the same identification number. It is important that a unified system be in place plant wide (or in some cases division wide) to identify pilot plant equipment and production equipment.

4. Day and Date of Work Performed

A standard format of recording the day and date of worked performed will help to eliminate miscommunication. The use of military time (such as 1400 hours for 2:00 PM) may be preferential in some environments where product and process are on a well-defined time continuum. The laboratory environments may work best in a month–day–year scenario. Computerized systems should be reviewed to assure all systems are date coding in a consistent fashion. In addition, the new millennium will add another dimension to the year portion of dating.

5. Location of Work Performed

Multiple sites within a division or corporation may carry the corporate distinction. A reviewer may not be able to distinguish data from individual sites if a secondary designation is not incorporated into the data-gathering process. One simple approach is to have the street address incorporated into all official data-recording documents. This can include individual laboratory notebook pages, individual data forms, all pages associated with the batch record, and individual logbook pages. This incorporation can be by design (a procedural requirement to have all official forms include an address header) or default (the use of an address stamp on all original pieces of documentation). Another advantage to this type of tracking system is an audit trail for the return of documents to their rightful owner if they are separated from the body of work.

6. Signature Lines

All original data collection tools will have a signature line for the originator and a witness or verifier. The space allotted to these lines vary as much as the penmanship of the person using the line. It is advisable to have a signature log in place for areas with the highest product impact, including laboratory, manufacturing, and filling environments. The signature log should include a place for full signature, initials, and a printed version of the person's legal name. This tool is invaluable when reviewing a body of work that spans many years.

As data are generated, the question of storage location becomes important. The overall body of work may be spread over several facilities and it may be impractical to store it physically as one unit. The FDA is charged in their Inspectional Guideline to verify the authenticity of the raw data that support the application. It is important to structure an "on-demand" retrieval system to meet an auditors/reviewers requests.

D. Recording of Data

Recording of data is an ongoing process during the lifetime of development of the product/process. Multiple schools of thought exist on how best to accomplish this task. A review of some of the most common methods of data recording illustrates the positive and negative aspects of each method.

1. Bound Versus Unbound Laboratory Notebooks

Bound notebooks offer a security advantage because pages cannot be removed without damaging the integrity of the volume. They can also open the door for a reviewer to venture beyond the scope of the original investigation if the notebooks are used for more than one product.

2. Electronic Data

Paperless systems offer the optimum in record-retention capacity. More data can be stored in less space by using paperless systems. They are also environmentally friendly by reducing the tonnage of paper used to record pertinent data. The challenge they provide is in security and validation. Data are more portable (data can be downloaded onto diskettes and removed without detection) and may be changeable depending on the security level attached to individual users.

3. Individual Batch Records and Stability Data

The individual batch record is a summary of the activities that account for the manufacture, filling, and testing of a product. These may be stored together as a single unit or maintained by each department. The raw material and component test records supporting the individual batch record may be stored by raw material or component part number or by lot number of the raw material or component. Stability data may be added to the individual batch record or stored by year or by product. Copies may be made of all of the original records and then forwarded to a central batch record folder to represent the individual batch record.

The advantage to storing the individual batch record and stability data for a single batch of product as one unit is the ease of reviewability and the ability to retrieve everything with one request. Individual storage units prevent the evaluation of the product as a whole.

4. Destruction of Data

In a perfect world, one would never need to destroy the data. However, the sheer volume of data requires that limits be set. The procedures governing record retention practices should be reviewed to determine if the potential exists to destroy submission data before the full approval of the application. It is especially important to assure that biobatches (batches of product used to support regulatory submissions and/or bioequivalency studies) are archived in a fashion that prevents their destruction for as long as the product in the market place.

5. Transferring Data Between Locations

Day-to-day systems may provide for the ongoing storage of data, but eventually, the data must be collected to support the application during an inspection. This may require the transfer of original data to a central location or the provision of equivalent review sites at each location of data generation. Centralization of data is optimal because it reduces secondary sites' exposure to additional FDA inspection and facilitates the review process. The risk is that data will not return to the site after completion of the review.

A well-organized plan of record retention/retrieval that anticipates these types of issues is an invaluable tool in preserving the audit trail of the technology transfer process.

IV. TECHNOLOGY TRANSFER MASTER PLAN: ELEMENT TWO— TECHNICAL WRITING STYLES

Internal audiences for the written word change as the product or process travels through the technology transfer cycle. The external audience is, by definition, the FDA. An overall awareness of the current audience and the final audience will help technical data generators build reports that accurately and effectively convey the details of the product or process.

It is important that the reader of any report clearly understand the conclusions or recommendations of the report. Effective technical writing styles have four common ingredients: (1) they accurately communicate the facts; (2) they keep the audience in mind; (3) they can be assembled with other reports and form an organized and consistent overview of the product/process; and (4) they do not use supposing statements.

The inclusion of these elements in the standards established for report generation will help assure that all readers will draw the same conclusions or make the same recommendations as the reports author.

A. Communicating the Facts

Tables, charts, graphs, and spreadsheets are all tools used to present facts in technical reports. These can be viewed as roadmaps of the development and technology transfer processes. As with any roadmap, the appropriate legends and markings should appear on the "map" to orient the reader.

The following two example tables represent the same database. Table 1 is a tabular representation of three columns wide and four rows long. The meaning of each value in the table is unknown to the reader because the first row does not include a column description. Table 2 is the same table with column headers. Now the reader knows that the data in column one is representative of the lot number (of the batch of material). Column 2 represents the batch size in liters, and column three is the expiration date of the material.

The two tables say the same thing but have different meanings to the reader. It is important to include the appropriate legends to accurately convey the facts. A standard glossary of legend markings and abbreviations can be an appropriate tool to assure consistency. This type of tool can compensate for differences in the training levels of data generating personnel. If everyone is using the same legends, misunderstandings are minimized.

B. Keeping the Audience in Mind

Technical writers tend to present data at the level it was collected. Data gatherers may be working on multiple projects and may record raw data in a notebook in the order it was collected. The notebook may contain more than one project. Should the FDA review this notebook for project A, they may also get an opportunity to review any of the other projects contained within the notebook. This may not be in the best interest of the company. The data gatherer may not be aware of the exposure potential of this type of data recording practice. It may be appropriate for

Table 1 Example One: Batches Awaiting Test Results

ABC34	37850	11-95
12345	18925	12-96
12XYZ	7570	1-98

Table 2 Example Two: Batches Awaiting Test Results

Lot number	Batch size (L)	Expiration date
ABC34	37850	11-95
12345	18925	12-96
12XYZ	7570	1-98

the technology transfer master plan to limit the use of one notebook for each project rather than assign one notebook to each data gatherer.

A data analyst may collect those notebooks and re-assemble the data into a chronology of events to show the course of development. This summary may not be as detailed as the notebook pages themselves, but generally will contain references to where the original data is located. It will be important that these references are accurate. If an error is observed in the original data, it may have impact on any data summary derived from the original data. If no reference is used it will be impossible to gauge the impact of the discovered error. The traceability of summaries to original data and vice versa is a key element for all reviewers.

The lack of traceability may cast doubt onto the validity of the data generated. The FDA is instructed in their inspectional guideline to assure the accuracy of the data that is included in regulatory submissions. The FDA cannot meet their guideline requirements if the original data cannot be located.

It may be appropriate for the technology transfer masterplan to include "go/no-go" points early in the development process that review all data for 100% data integrity. This system would identify data deficiencies in a timely manner and allow for the repetition of experiments to correct these deficiencies.

If the 100% data integrity criteria was met, the project would at a "go" and development would proceed to the next step. If the audit results were a "no-go," the opportunity exists to repeat the required work and then proceed. It would not be in the company's best interest to receive a "no-go" from the FDA.

C. The Pyramid Effect of Report Generation

In the overall historical perspective, a pyramid exists for all data generated for a single product or process. The overall development plan can consist of many small pyramids that collectively represent the product and the proces. Collectively, all data may support a regulatory submission, the top of the pyramid. The pyramid effect is defined by the whole being greater than the sum of the parts (Figure 2).

Each descending level of any pyramid will contain more detailed information, moving from the general to the more specific and concluding with the raw data itself. Each ascending level will contain data summaries and may generally be distributed to a wider audience.

It is important to remember that the raw data ultimately supports many documents and that any nomenclature changes can have an effect on a reader's understanding of the product/process.

At times, it may be appropriate to create a key or legend to product-specific details to aid a reader in understanding. A review or audit at certain pyramid levels to assure consistency, clarity, and 100% data integrity may be incorporated into the technology transfer master plan.

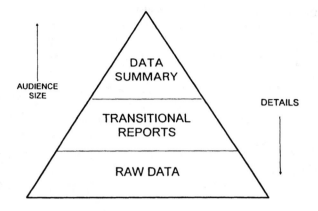

Figure 2   The pyramid effect of documentation.

D. Examples of Effective Writing Styles

As previously mentioned, technical writers tend to present data at the level it was collected. Without proper standardization, a data gatherer's previous training may be reflected in the manner in which data are recorded. The following three statement pairs illustrate this concept:

> *Statement Pair 1:*
> *"I thought my theory was correct, I think the data on page five proves it."*
> *"The theory was supported by the data generated on page 5."*
>
> *Statement Pair 2:*
> *"Analyst A must have recorded the boiling point in her notebook."*
> *"Analyst A recorded the boiling point of the liquid on page 25 of notebook 72."*
>
> *Statement Pair 3:*
> *"The batch records indicate that we should have used 100 liters of D water in Step 3."*
> *"Step three requires 100 liters of D water. The volume was recorded on page five of the batch record."*

The first statement in each pair uses personification. The tone of the statement casts doubt as to the validity of the data. The second statement in each pair is factual.

The use of personification should be discouraged during the course of data collection. The internal review of collected data should include a provision for the correction of personified data. A good rule of thumb when establishing review standards is: "If you aren't convinced, no one else will be either." It is important to remember that the company is the expert on the product and process. The FDA will review the data that are provided to them in a regulatory submission and all other support documentation required to determine the cGMP compliance status of the facility.

The use of supposing statements can be hazardous during the course of FDA review. These statements can cast doubt on the safety, purity, and efficacy of the drug product. Data should be dealt with as factual observations without personification. Investigations should contain facts with scientific judgement, quoting standard reference materials as appropriate. Reports should be comprised of facts, scientific judgement, and conclusions/recommendations.

V. TECHNOLOGY TRANSFER MASTER PLAN: ELEMENT THREE— ILLUSTRATION OF EQUIVALENCE

A. The Equivalency Concept

If "Location, Location, Location" is the key to a (great) real estate deal, then "Equivalence, Equivalence, Equivalence" is the key to technology transfer and scale-up. As a project progresses from conception to the bench, through the pilot plant, and eventually to production and commercial distribution, a series of technical modifications are performed. The overall goal in a technology transfer and scale-up master plan is to be able to trace and evaluate these modifications in a clear and understandable fashion.

The illustration of this equivalence is a key element of the reviewers audit program. The easier it is for a reviewer to see the equivalence modifications made to the product/process, the easier it will be for the reviewer to evaluate the change in regard to the safety, purity, and efficacy of the drug product.

Multiple options are available to illustrate equivalence. All of them are based on the adage: "A picture is worth a thousand words."

B. Side-by-Side/Step-by-Step Comparisons

Side-by-side/step-by-step comparisons are helpful when demonstrating the equivalence of different batch sizes for scale-up formulations. A simple block diagram can be generated, allocating one block for each step, assembling the steps in vertical order, and lining up each batch in size order. The steps can be as detailed as steps 1, 2, and 3 of a specific formulation, or as general as the manufacturing step, the packaging step, and the shipping step. This allows the reviewer to trace the steps horizontally as the batch is scaled up (Figure 3).

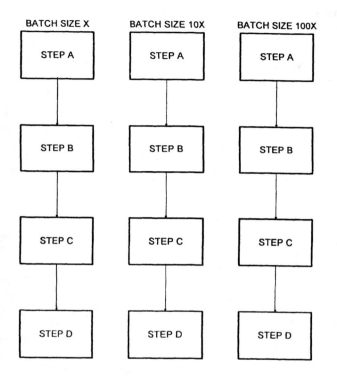

Figure 3 Side-by-side/step-by-step comparisons.

C. Flow Diagrams

Flow diagrams are tools for illustrating process modifications. One diagram can be made for each pivotal batch in the developmental process and then overlapped for comparison purposes. Additional narratives may be added to highlight the differences in the diagrams and for evaluation of the modification on the safety, purity, and efficacy of the product/process (Figure 4).

D. Critical Step Definitions

Critical step definitions are narrative comparisons of steps with the highest impact on the product/process that outline the operating parameters directly related to process control. They can be used in conjunction with flow diagrams to describe the product/process modification milestones in the technology transfer process.

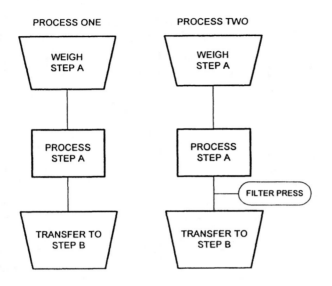

Figure 4 Flow diagrams.

E. Physical Space Comparisons

Physical space comparisons of tank, building, and filling equipment drawings are especially helpful when trying to illustrate environmental equivalence between different manufacturing facilities. Updated and verified site drawings of all research and production areas are excellent resources to obtain this information.

F. Terminology

Terminology equivalence is best achieved by the use of a glossary of standard terms. These can be agreed upon and modified as required during the course of product development.

VI. CONCLUSIONS

The overall goal for technology transfer and scale-up is to show, through process control, that any modifications made from conception to implementation have been appropriately evaluated and documented and that the product is safe, pure, and effective.

A well-organized plan that anticipates change is an invaluable tool in preserving the audit trail of the technology transfer process. A technology transfer master plan composed of three main components—documentation practices, technical writing styles, and the illustration of equivalence—can be used for any drug product or process. The tools outlined in this chapter can make the most complicated product/process easy to understand if they are used at the point of data generation.

10

Training of Personnel in the Pharmaceutical Industry

Tara V. Sams
Applied Analytical Industries, Inc. (AAI), Wilmington, North Carolina

I. INTRODUCTION

Training and the documentation of training is mandated by various pharmaceutical industry regulations and is likely to be reviewed during pre-approval inspections. Good Manufacturing Practice (GMP) regulations for the manufacture of pharmaceutical products as defined in the Code of Federal Regulations (CFR) state in Section 21 CFR 211.25 that each person shall have "education, training, and experience, or any combination thereof, to enable that person to perform the assigned functions," and that "training shall be in the particular operations that the employee performs" as well as in the "regulations themselves and written procedures required by the regulations as they relate to the employee's functions." Regulations state that training shall be "conducted by qualified individuals on a continuing basis and with sufficient frequency to assure that employees remain familiar" with the regulations applicable to them. In recent years there has been an increased emphasis on training programs and training documentation by the Food and Drug Administration (FDA) during their inspections of pharmaceutical firms. Common FDA citations for training violations include the following:

1. Lack of formal training documentation
2. Lack of training in GMP regulations on an ongoing basis
3. Lack of a formal job function training program
4. Lack of a system for evaluating and/or monitoring employees to ensure that training was effective

5. No provision for retraining individuals on a periodic basis to ensure that employees remain familiar with the requirements applicable to them
6. No provision for training employees on recently revised procedures
7. No provision for ensuring that employees were trained before performing job functions

In addition, many other FDA-cited violations also include adjunct citations for training deficiencies as a contributing factor for the cited violation.

Training programs should not, however, be developed merely to satisfy government regulations. Employees must have the knowledge and skills to perform the necessary job functions to achieve the company's goals. Remedial training may at times be required to correct deficiencies noted in employee performance, and cross-training can provide a more adaptable and flexible work force. Changes in technology, equipment and procedures, organizational focus, and other areas require that training be a continuous process and not just a one-time occurrence for new employees. Well-trained employees are more productive, produce better-quality science and documentation, and are more motivated and happier.

All company trainers should be well versed in contemporary adult training techniques. It is important to consider the background and level of education of the employees as well as their readiness to learn. Adult trainees must be motivated to learn by having an interest in the subject matter and an understanding of the need for the training and how it relates to their job responsibilities and career success. Adult trainees often benefit most from hands-on practice of techniques and principles of the training being conducted, which serves to further emphasize the applicability of the training. Trainers should be capable of maintaining leadership, creating an appropriate learning environment, controlling the group dynamics, and evaluating trainee comprehension.

Commitment and support of upper management is crucial to a successful training program. The coordination of training facilities, personnel, and operations must be managed. Good training programs take time and effort to develop and generally begin with a training assessment to determine training needs. Internally developed training programs require that appropriate personnel be given sufficient resources to develop training programs and related training materials, or alternatively, to evaluate external commercially available programs, seminars, consultants, or other resources.

An overview of several categories of training typically found in the pharmaceutical industry follows.

II. NEW EMPLOYEE ORIENTATION

New employee orientation training is typically performed the first week of a new employee's arrival.

Employees who are unfamiliar with the pharmaceutical industry can benefit from an overview of the pharmaceutical industry and the role their company plays in that industry. An overview of the pharmaceutical development process from discovery to commercial production is also helpful in allowing the employee to see how their job fits into the overall picture of pharmaceutical product development and production.

All employees can benefit from an overview of the company, including general mission and vision statements, long- and short-term goals, and general company policies. An overview of the company's organizational groups and their functions—including, if possible, work flow diagrams—is also helpful. This can be followed by departmental vision and mission statements and departmental goals, and how they fit into the corporate strategy. A specific job description for the employees should be provided, if available, including job performance requirements and goals. Most new employees also appreciate a tour of the company's local facilities, including all other departments as well as their own.

Company personnel policies are typically discussed with the employee during the first few days of employment. This overview routinely includes a discussion of administrative issues such as pay and benefits, work hours and absenteeism, performance appraisals, etc. Many companies also include a review of the company's Code of Ethics, to promote integrity and ethical practices and to prevent unethical or undesired conduct within the company.

Because of regulatory requirements, some basic safety training is also typically performed during the first few days of employment. Often, this safety training is required before the employee can work in the manufacturing or laboratory environment. Details of safety training are covered in Section IV.

Introductory regulatory training is often performed during orientation, particularly for employees inexperienced in the pharmaceutical industry. This training helps to prepare the new employee for the regulated work environment with its associated documentation requirements and provides an understanding and overview of the more detailed regulatory training to come later.

Temporary employees in the pharmaceutical industry may also require some formal training, particularly if they will be working in a position subject to regulations. This training is generally not as extensive as that for permanent employees, but may vary with the expected duration of employment and the level of supervision exercised.

III. REGULATORY TRAINING

All employees working in the pharmaceutical industry should be given training in the regulations that affect their jobs. This frequently includes Good Laboratory Practices (GLPs), GMPs, and/or Good Clinical Practices (GCPs). Introductory training in these regulations is normally performed during new employee orientation as defined above.

For more detailed training, a review of the appropriate regulations from the CFR governing the operations performed is a good place to start. Optimally, this is followed by a review of the company's standard operating procedures that define how the company specifically adheres to the regulations and the documentation practices used to ensure compliance. Because Food and Drug Regulations tend to be somewhat vague, specific examples of interpretation of the regulations should also be discussed. This may include FDA Guidelines and Inspection Guides, published industry guidelines, and/or examples of FDA 483 citations issued to the company or other companies. Training in internal quality controls and quality auditing procedures may also be included as part of this training. This allows the employee to know what to expect from internal quality monitoring procedures. Many companies also include training in dealing with FDA inspectors/investigators during regulatory training. This prepares all employees for handling questions during an FDA inspection.

GMP training for manufacturing and laboratory personnel is typically formalized, whereas technical support groups are often overlooked for formal job-specific GMP training. These groups should also receive GMP training specific to their job function. Technical support groups (or individuals) in need of formal GMP training might include the following:

1. Metrology or instrument calibration and maintenance groups
2. Computer or information systems departments
3. Document control and data archives groups
4. Data processing groups
5. Sample processing groups
6. Manufacturing warehouse management groups
7. Laboratory stockroom or stability storage personnel
8. Facilities maintenance
9. Training departments

Training in Drug Enforcement Agency (DEA) regulations must also be included for companies that handle controlled substances. This training should be performed for any research and development, manufacturing, laboratory, or support group that is involved in the handling or storage of controlled drugs. This training typically includes any required transfer paperwork, security procedures, inventory record keeping, and waste disposal required by DEA regulations.

Environmental Protection Agency (EPA) regulations as well as various local and state environmental regulations may affect many employees as well. Disposal of hazardous wastes, such as laboratory solvents, are subject to federal regulations under the Resource Conservation Recovery Act (RCRA), and most pharmaceutical waste and biohazardous waste treatment and disposal is regulated by various state and local agencies. For applicable employees, these regulations should be included as part of their formal regulatory training program.

IV. SAFETY TRAINING

All employees should be given training in general safety awareness, company safety rules (including any dress codes), and accident prevention. This training should include safety requirements for visitors and contracted service personnel.

Occupational Safety and Health Association (OSHA) requires that all employees exposed to potential chemical hazards be given training in "hazard communication." This training must include the location of material safety data sheets (MSDSs) and their use and interpretation. MSDS information generally includes the types of hazard(s), labeling requirements, safety precautions, and emergency procedures for the material being used. Any personnel who will be handling pharmaceutical materials that are toxic, carcinogenic, mutagenic, teratogenic, or highly potent compounds should be given specific training in the special handling of such materials, including the appropriate use of equipment (glove boxes, isolation or containment rooms, fume hoods, etc.) and the use of personal protective equipment and clothing. Specific decontamination and disposal procedures should also be discussed in detail.

Laboratory employees should also be given specific training in the appropriate handling, storage, personal protection, clean-up and decontamination, and disposal procedures for handling of hazardous chemicals (e.g., flammable solvents, corrosives, ethers, compressed gases) and biological fluids (potential bloodborne pathogens).

Exposure limits and personnel monitoring requirements that are part of the company's industrial hygiene plan should be discussed with applicable employees.

The use of personal protective equipment should be included in any safety training program. This may include the appropriate selection and use of gloves, respirators, face and eye protection, and protective clothing and shoes.

Generally, specialized training, including documentation requirements, should be given to any employee required to handle and dispose of waste materials classified as hazardous waste, pharmaceutical waste, or biological hazards.

Training in service maintenance hazards should be included for any employee who performs equipment repair and maintenance. This training includes the use of equipment guards, lockout/tagout training, protection from electrical hazards, etc.

Warehouse or other personnel who use forklifts, aerial lifts, or other industrial vehicles, as well as elevated equipment such as vertical extension ladders and scaffolds, should be trained in the safe use of this equipment.

All employees should receive training in emergency procedures. This includes location and operation of safety showers and eyewash stations, fire alarms, fire exits and evacuation routes, fire extinguishers, and emergency first aid kits. Reporting and documentation requirements for incidents and/or accidents should be included. This includes OSHA documentation requirements for reportable accidents and injuries.

V. JOB FUNCTION TRAINING

A. Research and Development Personnel

Research and Development personnel do not typically face the regulatory requirements for training that other departments must deal with; however, the FDA is beginning to look further into the development process than ever before, particularly during pre-approval inspections. Important decisions about the products developed are typically made during research and development, and there should be some assurance that the scientific systems used to develop and test these products in the early stages are reliable and thereby produce data for reliable and justifiable scientific decisions.

Inexperienced Research and Development personnel should receive training in research techniques and available technology specific to the products and processes being developed. Training in the use of specific equipment and instruments is generally included.

Documentation of scientific work is critical to the research and development process, as is the ability to retrieve this data at a later (often much later) date. Training in documentation techniques assures that thorough and appropriate scientific documentation is available and retrievable. This documentation may be critical during a pre-approval inspection for a new product, during technical transfers of technology to pilot plant and commercial manufacturing facilities, and for patent protection.

Validation of facilities, equipment, production processes, cleaning processes, computer systems, analytical methods, etc., is an area that receives much attention from the FDA. It is very important that personnel responsible for these activities receive complete and up-to-date training in the FDA's current expectations in this area. FDA guidelines are available and are updated periodically and multiple conferences and seminars in these topics are offered annually.

B. Production Personnel

Production personnel typically require job function training in materials control (including receiving, sampling, warehousing, and inventory control), in various production operations (including the operation of various manufacturing and packaging equipment), and in documentation practices.

Training in process control and quality control procedures should be included to ensure that all manufacturing personnel are familiar with control requirements.

Training in equipment set-up, cleaning, and/or maintenance, if production performs these functions, should also be included.

Specialized training in trouble-shooting and problem-solving techniques should be included for supervisory and other appropriate production personnel. This training typically also includes the investigation of product or process failures and required documentation.

C. Laboratory Personnel

New laboratory personnel typically receive training in general laboratory techniques (quantitative transfers, test method use, etc.), specific technical techniques to be used (high-performance liquid chromatography, gas chromatography, dissolution, etc.), and documentation and review practices. Investigation and reporting of aberrant or out-of-specification data should be included in the training program.

As in production, specialized training in trouble-shooting and problem-solving techniques should be included for supervisory and other appropriate laboratory personnel.

D. Technical Support Personnel

Technical support personnel are often overlooked in establishing formal training programs, both for regulatory and job function training. Job function training for these groups should minimally include: (1) operation of required instruments, equipment, and computer systems; (2) overview of applicable standard operating procedures; and (3) documentation practices.

E. Quality Control/Quality Assurance Personnel

Quality Assurance (QA) and/or Quality Control (QC) personnel should have formal training in the job functions they perform. This may include sampling and release of materials, quality review of documentation (standard operating procedures, specifications, test procedures, batch records, etc.), auditing and investigation techniques and documentation, and trending of quality data.

If vendor or contractor auditing is part of the QA/QC department's responsibilities within the company, training should be provided in appropriate auditing procedures and evaluation systems.

Most QA personnel also interact with regulatory agencies during inspections and should receive specialized training in how to handle such inspectional authorities.

E. Special Skills

Some special skills training is usually required in any pharmaceutical company, but the types of special skills needed may vary from company to company. The following are common examples of special skills training programs.

Scientific professionals sometimes lack the scientific writing skills that are vital to good communication of scientific results, particularly for research work. Verbal communication and presentation skills, particularly for supervisory and management positions, are also useful.

Computer skills are increasingly important in most pharmaceutical companies, and computer literacy is a requirement for many jobs, from secretarial and clerical staff to executive management.

Foreign language skills are valuable if the company is multinational or requires international travel.

VI. ADMINISTRATIVE TRAINING

As in any industry, the pharmaceutical industry should not omit administrative skills training from their formal training program.

Training in human resource issues can help employees understand governmental and company policies, provide enhancement of employee's personal growth, and provide a more well-rounded, healthy, productive employee. Stress management, time management, problem solving, work place ethics, dealing with conflict, sexual harassment, cultural diversity awareness, teamwork training, training skills, and communication skills are examples of beneficial training in this category.

Supervisory and management skills training are often needed for new supervisors and managers, as well as seasoned employees in some instances. Training in conducting interviews, leadership, motivating subordinates, disciplinary action, performance reviews, etc., is necessary.

Project Management is another area in which training can provide better organization for accomplishment of company goals. This training minimally includes formation of project teams, the use of planning and control tools, scheduling, budgeting, and project status communication.

VII. DOCUMENTATION OF TRAINING

Almost all training should be documented. Many regulatory agencies, including the FDA and OSHA, require documentation of employees' credentials in the form of training, education, and/or experience, and may request to see this documentation during routine inspections. Typically, these records are kept separate from other personnel records (such as those containing salary information or performance reviews) that are not inspected by regulatory agencies.

As a first step all employees should be required to have on file a current curriculum vitae that outlines a summary of their education and experience. These summaries should include details that describe their abilities to perform their current job function.

The training policies and documentation systems for the company should ideally be defined in standard operating procedures. These procedures should define the responsibilities for training activities, the requirements for internal trainer qualifications, the documentation of training, and the storage and archiving of training documents.

The training curriculum for each department's positions should be defined and monitored to ensure that each employee has received the appropriate training for their position. Generally, this curriculum includes company orientation training, applicable regulatory training, safety training, and training specific to the various job function(s) the employee will be performing, including operation of any equipment and documentation practices.

Monitoring may be the responsibility of the supervisor, the Training Department, an internal auditing group, or other appropriate personnel.

The qualifications of any internal trainers should be documented and maintained. Generally, these qualifications should indicate that the trainer has the necessary credentials to perform the designated training. A curriculum vitae or resume may be acceptable if credentials related to the training to be conducted are sufficiently detailed. If not, a "Trainer Certification Record" can be generated, detailing the qualifications of the trainer that are specifically related to the training to be performed. Any consultants used for training purposes should have their credentials on file as well.

Training records of regulatory and job function training should be maintained and should include the date of training, name of trainer and/or sponsoring organization, subject covered, exercises taken to ensure trainee comprehension, and certification of satisfactory completion of training by the trainer/organization.

Periodic updates of training and remedial training should be documented in addition to initial training.

VIII. PREPARATION FOR PRE-APPROVAL INSPECTIONS

Even if good training and training documentation programs are in place, most employees can still benefit from a pre-approval inspection preparation workshop. A list of the facilities, equipment, and documentation likely to be reviewed during the pre-approval inspection can be assembled and reviewed in advance for completeness. Any anomalies or problems that occurred during the product development should have adequate investigation reports, and any required follow-up actions should have been completed. Questions and concerns that are likely to be by raised by the FDA should be discussed in advance so that complete, clear, and adequate responses are prepared.

IX. CONCLUSIONS

Compliance with pharmaceutical industry regulations require that training be conducted and documented on a periodic basis. Good training programs are also necessary to ensure that employees have the knowledge and job skills required to function effectively and contribute to company objectives and goals, including successful pre-approval inspections. The support of upper management is critical to the success of any training program to ensure that adequate resources are provided for the planning, organization, and administration of training programs.

BIBLIOGRAPHY

1. Code of Federal Regulations, Drug Enforcement Administration, Department of Justice, 21 CFR 1300-1316.
2. Code of Federal Regulations, Clinical Investigations, 21 CFR 52.
3. Code of Federal Regulations, Good Laboratory Practices, 21 CFR 58.

4. Code of Federal Regulations, Good Manufacturing Practices, 21 CFR 210-211.
5. Code of Federal Regulations, OSHA Training Guidelines, 29 CFR 1910 and 1926.
6. G. Mitchell, *The Trainer's Handbook: The AMA Guide to Effective Training*, 2nd Edition, Amacom (American Management Association), New York, 1993.
7. W. R. Tracey, *Designing Training and Development Systems*, 3rd Edition, Amacom (American Management Association), New York, 1992.
8. *Training and Recordkeeping: OSHA/EPA/DOT Crossreference Manual*, J. J. Keller & Associates, Neenah, Wisconsin, 1995.

11

Compliance with Current Good Manufacturing Practices and Application Commitments

Anthony C. Celeste
AAC Consulting Group, Inc., Bethesda, Maryland

I. THE APPLICATION OF CURRENT GOOD MANUFACTURING PRACTICES TO THE DEVELOPMENT PROCESS

A. Background

The requirements of the Current Good Manufacturing Practice (CGMP) regulations regarding the development and preparation of investigational new drugs (INDs) for human use have recently been the topic of much discussion at the Food and Drug Administration (FDA). While the Agency has not fully determined what is required as CGMP for the development and production of clinical suppliers, it has opened the topic for discussion in a variety of forums and has taken regulatory action against at least one large contract producer of clinical supplies for inadequate CGMPs.

B. Clinical Supplies

An IND product for human use is defined as a drug product covered by an IND product application. These products, commonly referred to as clinical supplies, include the biobatch and pivotal study batches as well as all other drug products prepared for clinical trials. An underlying concern is the fact that product specifications and production methods for an investigational product may be subject to frequent change as the clinical testing of the product progresses.

The FDA recognizes that manufacturing procedures and specifications will change as clinical trials advance.

While recognizing the differences between the manufacture of investigational products and commercial products, the FDA has stated that it is vital that investigational products be manufactured under strict controls in conformance with CGMPs (2). Product contamination and wide variations in potency can produce substantial levels of side effects and toxicity, and can even produce wide-sweeping side effects on the physiological activity of the drug.

Product safety, quality, and uniformity are especially significant in the case of investigational products. Such factors may influence the outcome of a clinical investigation, thereby potentially affecting whether the product will be approved for wider distribution.

C. The Imposition of CGMPs

Aside from the CGMP issue, an IND study will not be allowed to proceed unless the reviewers at the FDA headquarters are satisfied that company drug development records adequately define the chemical, establish general safety, provide promise of efficacy, and document the ability to produce a product of acceptable quality. FDA investigators may be assigned to review development data. Usually such assignments are issued under the Good Laboratory Practices (toxicology laboratory) Program. When Agency personnel believe there are missing links in the documentation chain, the road to approval can be rocky. Over the years, researchers have complained that excessive documentation and maintenance of quality programs stifle the innovative process. Although there is some up-front time lost in following well-conceived, written, good development practice, quality assurance, or other such systems, that time is quickly recovered when work must be repeated or questions come from regulatory officials.

When, in the research and development (R&D) of a new drug, must a manufacturer comply with the provisions of the CGMP regulations? During initial research and development, there is experimentation with the new drug substance and its dosage form. Such experiments typically involve the drug's chemistry and toxicity studies conducted on laboratory animals. The CGMP regulations do not apply to the preparation of the new drug substance or drug products used in the initial preclinical experimentation that are not for human or, in the case of animal drugs, for therapeutic use.

When drug development reaches the stage at which the drug substance and products are produced for clinical trials in humans, then compliance with the CGMPs is required. The drug product must be produced in a qualified facility using qualified laboratory methods and equipment; the formula and process must be approved; manufacturing steps must be documented; records must receive appropriate reviews; and production processes must use qualified equipment and practices.

All manufacturing steps should be verified and checked; all appropriate in-process samples should be collected and analyzed; and documentation of all analytical procedures should be reviewed to ensure completeness as well as accuracy. Clinical batches should not be released until after the Quality Control (QC) unit has given its approval.

D. CGMP Compliance

The level of quality assurance (or CGMP compliance) for clinical batches should be equivalent to that for commercial batches. The expectation of the FDA is that firms have appropriate CGMP controls in place for manufacturing and QC operations. In general, "appropriate" means that validation should be performed to the extent feasible and that documentation of production and control may be less formal, but just as rigorous, as that for commercial products. The following sections clarify the FDA's expectations.

1. Research and Development Phase

Firms should expect FDA investigators to review the data used to support clinical trial batches to determine at which point CGMP controls were imposed and the decision made to produce clinical batches. This review may cover data as far back as the point when the firm decided that the active chemical (New Drug Substance) has pharmaceutical use. The FDA investigators' review covers standard operating procedures (SOPs) applicable to clinical supply production for completeness and appropriateness, with close attention to CGMP and documentation requirements. If no SOPs exist, the firms' actual practices may result in extra scrutiny by the FDA investigator.

Good documentation at these early product development stages will provide an excellent base for producing a product development report. Product development reports, while not required by the FDA, assist in the transition from R&D to production of the commercial drug product and identifies critical control points and parameters for process validation.

2. SOPs

During the IND stage of drug development, written production and control procedures are developed. Initially, these procedures may be more general as the procedures and controls are usually undergoing considerable refinement.

However, initial procedures should be as complete and detailed as knowledge and experience with the product and dosage form permit. These initial procedures must be reviewed and approved by the appropriate personnel (e.g., QC unit, production, laboratory) before implementation. Proper procedures must be followed and documented at the time of performance. Actual specific process control procedures and conditions such as timing, temperature, pressure, and adjustments (e.g., mixing, filtration, drying) should be fully documented to permit review and approval by the QC unit and to permit the development of more specific written production and control procedures as R&D reach conclusion. Additionally, all changes from initial procedures should be fully documented and based on well-founded scientific data or expert knowledge.

Written procedures for the general operation of the facility—including those for sanitation, calibration, and maintenance of equipment—and specific instructions for equipment use and procedures used to manufacture the drug product should also be in place.

3. Manufacturing and QC Systems

FDA investigators typically review manufacturing and QC records for record-keeping, component control, and in-process and final release testing. Although phase 1 clinical batches may be reviewed by the Agency, the investigators concentrate on the clinical supplies for later phases of clinical studies. Emphasis is more likely to be placed on the production and controls for phase 3 supplies.

4. Process Validation

At early clinical stages (phase 1 and phase 2) where a single batch of a drug product may be produced and where significant formulation and processing changes may make batch replication difficult or inexact, only limited process validation may be possible. In such cases, validation, especially for such critical processes as sterilization, should be derived from product and process analogs to whatever extent possible. In addition, data obtained from extensive process controls and intensive product testing may be used to demonstrate that the instant run produced a finished product meeting all of its specifications and quality characteristics. As additional uniform batches are made under replicated conditions, it is expected that more comprehensive process validation studies will be conducted.

At later development stages, such as phase 3 testing where multiple batches are created, more extensive process validation may be performed. At this stage, the FDA expects the equipment used to be qualified as to performance. Critical processes, including sterilization, aseptic fill, and environmental controls, must be fully validated. Each repetitive batch should meet the established product specifications (recognizing that these specifications may change). At this stage, it is very important that the actual process used is documented so that it can be duplicated.

During production for use in treatment INDs, the FDA's expectation is that process validation be underway, including an adequate validation plan with milestones. Some treatment INDs have progressed to extended studies with multiple batches. In these cases, the FDA expects that the validation studies be approaching completion and the sponsor have the following: (1) documentation for the validation studies underway and completed; (2) valid justification for any portion(s) of the studies not completed; and (3) established testing and process controls to ensure batch uniformity and conformance with predetermined specifications.

5. Product Specifications

The FDA recognizes that the experimental nature of the drug substance formulation and dosage form at an early stage of development impacts on establishing specifications. At early stages, the acceptance/rejection criteria may not be as clearly defined. However, it is vital that such acceptance/rejection criteria be scientifically sound and based on available scientific data. Specifications used as the basis for approval or rejection of components, containers, and closures will be more specific and uniform as additional data become available. At all stages, it is vital that specifications used are fully documented. Significant differences between actual and theoretical yields can signal processing errors that result in mix-ups, superpotency, subpotency, and contamination. Therefore, it is essential to reconcile those differences.

In the case of INDs, a variety of factors, including the preparation of relatively small batch sizes and the subdivision of in-process material for research purposes, may result in significant yield discrepancies. These resulting discrepancies do not necessarily imply problems; however, yield discrepancies must be evaluated because other potential factors may have induced the discrepancies and may signal processing errors. Specifications regarding theoretical yield that would trigger an investigation may initially be wider than at later stages of the product's development. Nonetheless, it is vital that those initial specifications be established using the best information available and adequate in-process controls to ensure a final product that meets the specifications of strength, identity, and purity.

As clinical investigations progress and experience with production of the product increases, the FDA expects that these specifications will narrow and reach levels that will be appropriate for full-scale commercial production. Where yield discrepancies are significant or unexplained, it is essential that products not be released unless, and until, there is reconciliation of all materials used at each appropriate phase of production and other appropriate investigations have been conducted.

In summary, CGMPs apply to all drug products intended to be administered to humans. The FDA expects that manufacturers have SOPs for production and control procedures, as well as for critical processes such as sterilization and aseptic fill. For these critical processes, the Agency also expects limited validation to be completed. This limited validation may be based on data from other products and processes as well as on specific installation qualification and process validation studies.

II. IMPORTANCE OF GOOD DOCUMENTATION AND SYSTEMS

Unfortunately, because of the work it takes to reorganize or to revise procedures, many companies are operating under procedures and systems that have become a patchwork quilt. Frequently, firms' documentation includes redundant or overlapping procedures and active documents that are obsolete in view of actual practices. Poorly managed total quality management (TQM) and continuous quality improvement (CQI) programs, as well as overreaction to the many FDA GMP inspection guidelines, have resulted in prevention programs being added to outmoded QC-oriented structures. Flawed quality systems can allow surprising failures and undetected defects that result in unnecessary rework or recall expenditures.

The bottom line is that all development laboratories should have basic quality assurance programs whether or not they intend to conduct research that could become part of a submission to a regulatory agency. While there are no CGMP regulations that are directly applicable when a substance is undergoing only in vitro studies, it is reasonable that the FDA would expect good practice to be followed in producing the study drug. A quality assurance program that includes the basics discussed in this chapter is a practical necessity.

A. Documentation of Operations and Controls

Pharmaceutical manufacturing operations and corresponding QC and quality assurance systems are required by regulation to be managed under a relatively large number of written procedures. The general requirements for documentation are the same as those set forth in the International Organization for Standardization ISO 9000 quality standards, Military Standard MIL-Q-9858A, and other quality systems guidances. The FDA CGMP regulations and guides for interpreting the regulations for different classes of products specify the rigor of control for certain operations and directly or indirectly mandate certain written procedures. Well-developed procedures for product development, manufacturing, and postmarketing activities (1) facilitate management of operations and quality systems; (2) improve communications and guidance; and (3) assure consistent and complete performance of assigned tasks.

B. Defining the Written Procedure

It is important to note that the CGMPs do not define what constitutes a written procedure, nor do the rules differentiate between written procedures prepared as SOPs and those prepared as detailed instructions in the master production and control records. The rules require that there be a written procedure for the preparation of master records; therefore, it would appear that written procedures that are commonly referred to as SOPs are the foundation of the documentation systems. Accordingly, one or more SOPs should authorize, define, and set forth controls for all subordinate document systems such as master records, batch production records, bills of materials, analytical records, engineering drawings, forms, etc. As a practical matter, the regulations only require that written procedures be understood and followed, and neither the format nor the type of document used is important unless the system fails.

Certainly, many written procedures should be prepared and kept current beyond those specifically required by the regulations. A rule of thumb is to write a procedure for operating or controlling each piece of equipment, system, or process that must be calibrated, maintained, qualified, or validated. Some FDA officials have said that whenever a qualifier appears in the CGMPs such as "suitable," "adequate," or "appropriate," a procedure must be written to set forth the detail, frequency, or other aspects of the control.

In large manufacturing facilities involving many people of various skill levels, well-organized and managed written procedures are always necessary. In a small firm, communication lines are usually short, few people are involved, and management is readily available to provide guidance so that written procedures may be less comprehensive than those for a large firm and still meet minimum CGMP requirements. A firm, particularly a small firm, may conclude that the specific language of the regulation for certain written procedures is not directly applicable to specific operations. However, such decisions must be documented and demonstrated a valid alternative control is present to meet the objective of the required written procedure.

It is also important to understand the utility of the many Inspection Guides that are being published by the FDA. These documents are written primarily for the FDA's internal use as training materials and/or to promote consistency in approach to inspections by the many FDA field offices. Some of these guides have not been updated for a number of years and contain some outdated information. The guides are not regulations and are merely interpretative documents. Most of them contain a disclaimer that they do not bind the FDA or convey any rights or privileges on any person. Nevertheless, they are a source of background material when first preparing a new procedure.

Companies must evaluate each of their operations and determine the need for written procedures based on the training and knowledge of the operators and the control needed to meet specifications. If reprocessing, rework, confusion, or complaints suggest that unsafe or ineffective products are likely to be or are being distributed, then written procedures for control, investigation of cause, and other corrective actions are clearly needed. Written procedures and associated manufacturing and control records should define all activities required to operate in a state of control and describe the documentation required to confirm that they have been performed. Such procedures should provide for verification of critical manufacturing operations. Diagrams, blueprints, illustrations, photographs, etc., are often used to supplement written procedures. The caliber of training programs and the work experience of employees may be considered in determining the detail necessary in a specific written procedure. For example, machinists are typically skilled personnel who fabricate components and finished devices using dimensioned drawings for guidance instead of written procedures.

C. Developing Procedures

Many firms should consider restructuring their documentation control systems to better accommodate a growing number of procedures or to improve their ability to electronically cross-reference, retrieve, and control procedures. In a comprehensive review of a quality system, areas needing written procedures may be identified by carefully examining production and laboratory operations in the following areas (consolidated from the CGMPs and ISO 9000):

1. management responsibility
2. quality system structure and procedures control
3. product development
4. product formulation or design
5. validation of test methods
6. purchasing and materials control
7. qualification, calibration, and maintenance of equipment
8. process design and validation
9. in-process controls, including identification of equipment and materials
10. training and supervision of employees
11. master and production records control
12. recording of test and inspection data
13. failure, deviation, and out-of-specification investigations
14. storage, distribution, and traceability

15. complaint reporting, evaluation, and follow-up
16. internal audits and product reviews
17. any other activity related to the quality of the product

An aide to the development of written procedures is flowcharting, which includes the step-by-step charting of the minute details of each operation. Internal and external audit reports are also very helpful in determining what is actually happening in particular operations. Audit findings can be noted on flow charts or otherwise cross-referenced. The knowledge gained from both flowcharts and audit reports will help identify potential manufacturing and quality problems.

From a company personnel management viewpoint, the reason for studying and charting a given activity should be discussed beforehand with affected personnel. Their input should be requested with respect to assuring the proper level of detail. By using the information presented in a flowchart and the experience gained developing a chart, production, engineering, quality assurance, and documentation personnel are better able to: (1) analyze the particular operation with respect to process requirements; (2) determine what needs to be added, modified, or deleted to solve any problems or improve performance; and (3) as appropriate, write or modify a procedure to cover a new way of performing the activity.

D. Addressing Specific Needs

Investigations of incidents of employee confusion, equipment malfunctions, process failures, rework, and customer complaints may lead to the discovery of inadequate process design/validation or QC deficiencies. Such inadequacies may involve components, equipment, maintenance, operation techniques, documentation, and environment. A written procedure may alleviate a systemic problem; however, the cause must be corrected before an adequate document can be written.

Developing written procedures generally consumes a considerable amount of both operational and management time in all affected departments. This sometimes results in "back-of-the-envelope" notes and uncontrolled memoranda being written instead of formal procedures. Likewise, changing procedures is time-consuming, and the need to meet production deadlines or lack of available personnel may result in forgetting to make necessary changes. Recording and monitoring all proposed changes to closure is therefore necessary.

It is important to develop written procedures that are concise, clear, and designed to prevent problems. Users of procedures, including new employees that are provided minimum training, must be able to understand and follow the directions. All employees and management personnel should be encouraged to submit proposals for new or revised procedures that will improve production and quality management systems. Some businesses offer financial incentives to reward suggestions that are accepted. A form is often used to identify the problem or potential problem to be addressed, and a proposal or a draft of the suggested new procedure or revision is submitted.

The same form or another method may be used to record decisions on whether a recommended new or modified procedure is needed. Other records may be used to obtain input from affected departments on whether the procedure is needed and, if so, their comments. In some instances, it may be determined that the existing procedure is adequate and that training should be improved or the number of trained back-up personnel should be increased.

The mechanics of drafting or changing written procedures can introduce errors; therefore, manufacturers are encouraged to use computers in writing, archiving, and changing procedures. These tasks become easier with computers; however, security must be maintained and archives protected.

E. Format of Procedures

Experience with quality systems management in the FDA-regulated industries has shown that procedures should contain the following header information:

1. company identification
2. title that reflects the activities to be performed
3. identification or control number with a revision level code
4. effective date
5. the number of pages in the procedure (e.g., 1 of 4)
6. approval date and signature(s)

The effective date may be the same as the final approval date; however, some firms delay effective dates to afford for training employees on the new procedures. All required departmental signatures and approval dates may appear on a separate document such as a QC change order or document control form. The main body of the procedure should cover the following, as appropriate:

1. subject, scope, objectives (including problem alerts)
2. references to related procedures, instructions, or forms
3. who has responsibility for performing each task
4. what activity or task is to be performed
5. when and where the task is to be performed
6. how to perform the task, including what tools, materials, etc., to use.

Background information helps employees to understand an assignment and remember how to perform it. Particularly for the new employee, it is important that the procedure concisely state the reason for performing a function and why it must be performed in a certain way. Employees working in environmentally controlled, clean manufacturing areas need to be aware of invisible microbes and particulates, and that humans are a major source of these unwelcome contaminates. If informed, employees are more likely to follow the operational procedures for working in controlled areas.

The task description in each procedure should cover appropriate details such as the following:

1. concise step-by-step instructions
2. the expected results from performing the tasks
3. where to place equipment or materials
4. what data to collect and how to analyze, file, and/or report
5. any related activities that need to be performed for the overall operation to remain in a state of control or for the product to meet all of the master record specifications.

F. Document Change Control

Procedures change control is an area that is often overlooked as businesses grow, reorganize, and restructure operations. A well-conceived system for managing the documents that control operations and quality functions will afford control over the manufacturing practices themselves. We have seen many different document change control systems that work well. Some are resource-intensive and involve a large documentation staff. Others are highly computerized and allow the rapid search of procedures by department, function, equipment, product, process, etc.

Because forms are frequently printed and stocked in large quantities in central areas, it is desirable to identify and control forms separately from procedures. Forms can be issued and changed as attachments to procedures; however, this usually wastes paper and burdens the procedure distribution process. However they are controlled, procedures and instructions should direct the use of forms and the information to be recorded. When a document must be revised, the document change control system should identify all related procedures, instructions, and forms that should be considered for a corresponding revision.

The importance of change control can be illustrated, e.g., with a pharmaceutical company that is replacing all glass containers with plastic containers. The procedures being developed should cover the clearing of the new packaging lines, maintenance and calibration of equipment, and instructions for operators. An existing qualification procedure should be followed to assure proper functioning of the new equipment. With so many ongoing activities, one must wonder if the change control system will assure attention to related activities such as changes to master records, labeling specifications, and New Drug Application (NDA)/Abbreviated NDA (ANDA) submissions. If not, the finished drug product may not meet the requirements of the GMP regulations or approved NDA/ANDA commitments.

After a procedure is developed, before final approval and implementation, it should be reviewed with the affected personnel. If necessary, a formal training course or program should be conducted for the affected personnel. During the initial implementation, the use of the procedure should be monitored closely. After gaining experience using the procedure, fine-tuning is often necessary, and the document should be changed (using the change control system) to more exactly meet the needs of the operation or process. This should be made clear in the written procedures governing change control because many persons are reluctant to promptly initiate second change and will continue to use a flawed procedure.

Finally, it should be noted that well-managed documentation systems are not without costs. It is commonly known that satisfactory documentation of a quality system to one of the ISO 9000 Quality Standards is the greatest barrier to registration. The "current good" aspect of CGMP requires that procedures be reviewed and that updating be considered on a regular basis. Most drug firms have procedures on a 1- or 2-year review cycle. When an FDA investigator or an ISO auditor sees a number of procedures that have not been updated for a number of years, he or she will immediately begin to question the quality system.

III. IMPLEMENTATION OF APPLICATION COMMITMENTS

The Food, Drug and Cosmetic Act provides explicit authority for the FDA to refuse to approve NDAs, ANDAs, and Antibiotic Drug Applications (AADAs) if the methods used in, and the facilities and controls used for, the manufacture, processing, packing, and testing of the drug are inadequate to ensure and preserve its identity, strength, quality, and purity.

The applicant is required to submit information in the application to the Center for Drug Evaluation and Research (CDER), including details as to how the firm proposes to manufacture and control the manufacture of the active substance and of the dosage form (product). The application is reviewed by CDER scientists (chemists, microbiologists, etc.). The FDA districts (investigators, chemists, and, as appropriate, microbiologists) examine the adequacy of the firm's facilities from a CGMP standpoint and audit the information submitted in the application. The districts recommend approval or withholding of the application based on their evaluation of the firm's CGMPs and the firm's compliance with its application commitments.

The Pre-Approval Compliance Program is designed to provide close inspectional and analytical attention to the authenticity and accuracy of data in applications and information regarding facilities. Such coverage is necessary to assure applications are not approved if there are significant questions about the completeness and/or reliability of the application, the GMP compliance of the pre-approval batches, and the capability of the applicant to meet the application commitments.

Fraudulent practices in the generic drug industry discovered in 1989 made it clear that closer attention should be given to the data submitted in applications. Inspectional experience relative to these fraudulent practices revealed discrepancies between representations made in some ANDAs concerning manufacturing procedures, batch size, and formulations of batches used to conduct bioequivalence studies and the actual practices of the applicants. Additionally, there were instances in which the stability data submitted to the Agency were fraudulent.

To deter future similar incidents in applications, and to assure early detection should such incidents occur, the Agency instituted several measures:

1. The FDA expanded its inspection program beyond the required biennial on-site inspection obligation to include additional criteria for triggering inspections. Under this expanded program, firms may receive product-specific pre-approval inspection even though they may have been covered recently if the drug products: (1) have a narrow therapeutic range, such as drugs used to treat epilepsy, asthma, high blood pressure, and heart disease; (2) are among the top 200 most prescribed drugs; (3) are new chemical entities; and (4) represent a new dosage form product for the applicant. The FDA will also inspect applicants with a history of noncompliance with CGMPs and applicants who have not previously submitted an application.

2. The pre-approval program includes audits of the manufacturing and control records concerning batches used to conduct bioavailability, bioequivalency, and stability studies. Investigations have shown a number of instances in which the batches of a drug product used to conduct a bioequivalency study differed from the batches of the drug represented in the ANDA and subsequently marketed. In some cases, manufacturing procedures and/or formulations were different from those in the application. Adequate and accurate information in an application about the batches of drug used to conduct bioavailability, bioequivalence, and stability studies is crucial to the demonstration of bioequivalence of a generic drug product to the innovator's product, and to the demonstration of stability in any product.

3. Before any application is approved by the CDER, a determination will be made whether all establishments that will participate in the manufacture, packaging, QC, or testing of the finished dosage form or new drug substance are in compliance with the CGMPs and application commitments. This approval process has basically two components: (1) the scientific evaluation conducted by the CDER review divisions, based on the application; and (2) compliance evaluation

of the facilities identified in the applications, basically to determine whether they are in compliance with the law.

The objectives of the pre-approval inspections include the following:

1. evaluation of the establishment's compliance with CGMP requirements, including coverage of the specific batches used to support the application (e.g., biobatch, stability batches)
2. evaluation as to whether the establishment has adequate facilities, equipment, procedures, and controls to manufacture the product in conformance with application commitments
3. audit of the accuracy of the pre-approval batches' manufacturing and testing information submitted with the application
4. collection of forensic samples of the biobatch from the bioequivalence test laboratory and from the applicant
5. collection of methods validation or methods verification samples

Inspections are conducted in the following cases:

1. when the subject of applications are a narrow therapeutic range of drugs, new chemical entities, or generic versions of the 200 most prescribed drugs
2. when the manufacturing plant and/or dosage form has not had an acceptable inspection in the past two years
3. when the application is from a firm whose applications were the subject of a validity assessment
4. when the application is the initial one for the applicant
5. when the manufacturer of the substance has not already received a satisfactory GMP inspection or is producing a substance by a process that has not been previously inspected; the FDA will inspect the substance producer under this program
6. at CDER and/or district discretion

In addition to original NDA/ANDA applications, certain supplemental applications may be similarly covered. Certain types of INDs (e.g., treatment INDs) will also receive inspection.

A. Pre-Approval Compliance Evaluation

The CDER's Office of Compliance completes the compliance evaluation after considering all pertinent information, including district recommendations. They will recommend withholding approval when there are significant deviations from CGMPs or application commitments that may adversely impact on the product. The District may send a letter advising the plant officials (or sponsor when appropriate) that the district has recommended withholding of approval and the reasons for the recommendation.

If applications are withheld because of significant CGMP noncompliance, and the GMP deficiencies also apply to commercially marketed products, then action must be taken to assure that the deficiencies are corrected.

Applications will not be withheld for the lack of complete, full-scale, multiple-batch validation unless the data submitted in the application are found to be fraudulent. Although the Agency does not require the manufacturer to fully validate the manufacturing process and control procedures before approval, the CDER reviewers do require that certain data be filed to demonstrate that a plant's sterilization and aseptic fill processes have been qualified.

Companies must fully validate the production processes using the specifications listed in the filing. Because process validation is a significant part of the CGMPs and assuring the adequacy of the filed process, companies are expected to complete validation before shipment. Otherwise, the distributed product is deemed violative and subject to regulatory action (i.e., seizure). Post-approval inspections may be made from time to time to assure validation has been performed in an acceptable manner.

B. Responsibilities of FDA Field Office Versus the CDER

To fully understand the FDA's expectations with regard to application commitments, it may be appropriate to briefly overview the center and field responsibilities in this program area.

The Compliance Program on Pre-Approval Drug Inspections/Investigations (7346.832) has, for the past several years, been the major drug program used for inspections of drug manufacturers. This program, which outlines the roles of the CDER and the FDA field investigators in the drug approval process, has recently (1994) been completely revised. The revised version provides improved, more comprehensive guidance for all phases of pre-approval inspections, investigations, sample collecting, laboratory evaluations, and assessment of overall findings.

The CDER's role in the pre-approval process is to review data submitted to the Agency as part of premarket NDAs and generic drug applications, and establish specifications for the manufacture and control of the resulting drug product based on the submitted data. The CDER continues to evaluate test methods, specifications, and data generated from these methods for adequacy and appropriateness.

The field investigator audits the data and is responsible for determining the adequacy of the facility, personnel, and equipment qualification information during the CGMP portion of the inspection. The field investigator's role is to assure CGMP compliance, verify the authenticity and accuracy of the data contained in these applications, and report any other data that may impact on the firm's ability to manufacture the product in compliance with GMPs.

The cooperation between the CDER and FDA field investigators and the resulting benefit to the industry is the communication of clearer agency expectations in the pre-approval area. A firm should be well prepared for a comprehensive pre-approval inspection covering not only the production of the target product, but also extensive reviews of data covering procedures and validation of the process and ancillary systems (e.g., environmental controls, equipment qualification, personnel training, and change control). Firms should also be aware that contract manufacturers and producers of critical components, including the active substance(s), and new excipients may be inspected by the agency before approval.

The previous program did not explicitly define the roles of the FDA districts and the CDER. This led to some confusion and disagreements regarding the policies involved. Firms were occasionally given conflicting information from Agency sources. The current revision represents a great effort on the part of the Agency to define the respective unit roles by explicitly comparing the district objectives and responsibilities in conducting pre-approval inspections, compared with the responsibilities assigned to CDER scientists. The following sections discuss the different responsibilities.

1. Biobatch Manufacturing

District inspection to determine the establishment's compliance with CGMPs includes data audits of the specific batches on which the application is based (e.g., pivotal clinical, bioavailability, bioequivalence, and stability). Field investigators look for changes that have occurred between the manufacture of batches on which the application is based and the manufacture of commercial batches. Firms need to have supporting data for any changes in process that may result in product differences affecting bioavailability and/or bioequivalency.

CDER scientists/reviewers are responsible for the review and evaluation of the records and data submitted in the application, including the components, composition, batch instructions, in-process and finished product test points, and specifications established for the resulting drug product.

2. Manufacture of Drug Substances and Excipients

The district determines CGMP compliance of the establishment. CDER chemists are responsible for the scientific review and evaluation of the records and data associated with the manufacture of the active drug substance submitted in the application or a properly referenced Type II Drug Master File (DMF).

The manufacture of novel excipients may be provided for in an application or supporting DMF. Typically, these excipients are noncompendial and used in specialized dosage forms and drug delivery systems. CDER chemists are responsible for the scientific reviews and evaluation of the records and data associated with the manufacture of these novel excipients. The review will include starting materials, key intermediates, reagents, and solvents. CGMP inspections by the field investigator will be performed upon request from the CDER.

In their reviews, Agency personnel will generally use the following documents. CDER chemists will use the CDER "Guidelines for Submitting Supporting Documentation in Drug Applications for the Manufacture of Drug Substances." District investigators primarily use: (1) "Guide to Inspections of Bulk Pharmaceutical Chemicals"; and (2) "Guide to Inspections of Sterile Drug Substance Manufacturers."

3. Raw Materials (CGMP Controls)

The district inspects the establishment for the drug substance and reviews data on raw materials to determine compliance with Section 501 (a)(2)(B) and DMF requirements. These controls are evaluated in the plant by the field investigator as part of the CGMP inspection of the facility and are not required to be submitted to the application.

4. Raw Materials (Tests, Methods, and Specifications)

Districts audit the data submitted for CDER review in the application. CDER chemists are responsible for the scientific review of the associated data; evaluations of the adequacy of the submitted data; and the ultimate approval of the tests, methods, and specifications established for the raw materials in the application.

5. Composition and Formulation of Finished Dosage Form

Districts audit the data submitted for CDER review in the application. CDER reviewers are responsible for the scientific review of the composition and formulation to determine, qualitatively and quantitatively, the acceptability of the information submitted in the application.

6. Container/Closure System(s)

The CDER is responsible for the scientific review of the container/closure systems to be used to package the drug product as indicated in the application. Districts may audit these data and will ensure that no changes in material and/or packaging composition have occurred during scale-up to commercial lots.

7. Labeling and Packaging Controls

The district inspects to determine the establishment's compliance with CGMP requirements and audits the data submitted for CDER review in the application. (Note: there are new CGMP requirements for labeling controls.)

8. Labeling and Packaging Materials

The CDER reviewers are responsible for the scientific review of the labeling and packaging components associated with the drug product.

9. Laboratory Support of Methods of Validation

Upon CDER request, district field laboratory analysts will conduct laboratory validation of the analytical methods proposed by the applicant. CDER laboratories may participate in certain instances (AADA validations, etc.).

CDER chemists are responsible for the review and acceptance/rejection of the analytical methods based on the laboratory results and the established specifications. Contacts between field laboratory analysts and the applicant will include the CDER chemist.

10. Product (CGMP) Controls

The district inspects the establishment to determine compliance with CGMP requirements, and reviews and audits the data furnished to the CDER in the application. The CDER scientists will request information on sterile processes— e.g., laboratory controls for environmental monitoring, sterile fill operations, and evaluation and reduction of microbial contamination—to be submitted to the application for CDER review.

11. Product Tests, Methods, and Specifications

A field district investigator is responsible for auditing the data submitted for CDER review in the application. The CDER is responsible for the scientific review of the associated data and the ultimate approval of the tests, methods, and specifications established for the drug product in the application. The field investigator will advise the CDER when he or she finds a questionable specification.

12. Product Stability

The district inspects the establishment to determine compliance with CGMP requirements and the validity of data supporting product stability, and conducts an audit of the data furnished to the CDER in the application. This requirement applies to both the relevant pre-approval batches, as previously discussed, and the proposed commercial batches.

The CDER review chemists are responsible for the review of the proposed drug product stability protocol, specifications, and evaluation of the data submitted in support of the expiration dating period proposed for the drug product in the application.

13. Comparison of the Relevant Pre-Approval Batch(es) and Proposed Commercial Production Batches

CDER chemists are responsible for the comparison of the formulation, manufacturing instructions, and associated in-process and finished product tests and specifications established for the relevant pre-approval batch(es) with the proposed commercial production batch to determine the acceptability of the firm's proposed scale-up procedure.

Districts compare the process used to make the pre-approval batches with the *actual* process used to manufacture the validation batches. Significant differences in these processes are evaluated by the CDER's Office of Compliance to determine whether the differences are significant and whether any differences constitute fraud. The reviewing officers also determine whether differences in the processes will affect the safety and effectiveness of the resulting process.

14. Facilities, Personnel, and Equipment Qualifications

Districts review the information and inspection of the establishment to determine compliance with CGMP requirements. This will be evaluated in the plant by the field investigator as part of the CGMP inspection of the facility and is not required to be submitted in the application.

15. Equipment Specification(s)

Districts audit the data submitted for CDER review in the application. CDER scientists are responsible for the review of equipment specifications furnished to the CDER in the application.

16. Packaging and Labeling (CGMP Controls)

Districts review the CGMP controls and inspect the establishment to determine compliance with CGMP requirements. These controls are evaluated in the plant by the field investigator as part of the CGMP inspection of the facility and are not required to be submitted in the application.

17. Process Validation

Districts inspect the establishment to determine compliance with CGMP requirements and adherence to application requirements. The CDER may request data to support validation of sterile processing operations, e.g., environmental monitoring, equipment validation, sterile fill validation, and associated sterile operations.

18. Reprocessing

Districts inspect the establishment to determine compliance with CGMP requirements and conduct an audit of the data submitted to the CDER in the application. CDER application review chemists are responsible for review of reprocessing protocols proposed in the application. All reprocessing procedures must be validated and/or scientific data must be available to justify the reprocessing procedure. Districts audit the validation of these procedures.

19. Ancillary Facilities

Districts are responsible for the review of this information. Upon CDER request or in district management's judgment, ancillary facilities (contract labelers) will be inspected to determine compliance with CGMP requirements. The name, address, and function of each ancillary facility is required to be indicated in the drug application.

The CDER will review biological and immunological test methods and results submitted. The revision of the pre-approval compliance program in 1994 clarified the roles of CDER and the field investigators. Concurrently, a number of administrative actions have greatly increased the communication of the FDA field staffers and the CDER reviewers. A firm may find that the investigational team and the CDER chemists remain in contact throughout the period of the pre-approval inspection.

IV. THE INTERNAL AUDIT PROGRAM

Some time ago, an FDA field official spoke at an industry seminar and said that a good case could be made under existing CGMP rules that internal audit programs are mandatory. The only explicit GMP requirement for internal audit is in the medical device regulations (21 CFR 820). That field official's view apparently did not catch on because little more has been said. However, when experts testify as to what is CGMP in both products liability cases and civil and criminal cases brought by regulatory agencies, they are likely to state that audit systems are accepted in the pharmaceutical industry as current good practice. Certainly, defendants in such cases may have failed to exercise due diligence if they have no internal audit program.

At what level should internal audit programs be administered. The FDA's good manufacturing practices regulations require management of a company to assure that quality assurance programs are effective. While the level is not specified, the Agency makes it quite clear that quality decisions must be made by someone other than manufacturing or marketing personnel to avoid conflicts of interest. As previously discussed, the ultimate legal responsibility for product quality rests with the CEO and corporate management.

Occasionally, an FDA manager will state that corporate audit programs should be patterned after the FDA inspection program. Corporate audits should be superior to FDA inspections in many respects. Because of the law enforcement responsibilities of the FDA, it could not engage in a partnership aimed at quality improvement. The corporate audit frequency and depth should be more efficiently managed because the audit staff has one master to serve rather than the White House, Congress, consumer groups, etc., as does the FDA. Personnel with superior technical ability in a particular field can be assigned to audit positions and trained in audit techniques. They should be able to access information more easily than FDA investigators. Audit follow-up and problem-solving should be better focused and timely when legal constraints are removed.

Most major pharmaceutical companies have a corporate audit program that covers manufacturing operations. Some programs audit research activities as well. Most have a complete audit cycle of two years, with more frequent audits in the event of problems. A corporate official is generally responsible for the audit; however, many programs rely heavily on subordinate divisions to provide audit support. Some use audit teams composed of both corporate and subsidiary staff, delegate some of the on-site work, or use various combinations of both. Some companies with corporate audit programs also require each manufacturing or research site to have its own internal audit program. In the latter instance, the corporate and local audit groups frequently share their schedules and sometimes may even share their findings.

Departments or sites should have a clear understanding of the audit standards that will be used to evaluate their operations. Some companies have developed comprehensive standards of their own, whereas others rely on published documents such as the ISO Standards and or the FDA Inspection Guides. It is important to schedule the audits well in advance, provide the unit to be audited with a general audit plan, and not depart from the plan unless a significant deficiency must be explored. The latter will help assure that personnel are available to assist in providing information and documents to the auditors.

Common complaints about audit programs that should be addressed by management include the following:

1. The corporate auditors do not know enough about the controls necessary in businesses they are auditing.
2. The corporate audit does its thing without any regard to our local audit program or our schedules.
3. The program seems to compel our auditors to find something wrong even when things are really in good shape.

4. Corporate management incorrectly views all FDA investigator observations as "violations" (they are indeed listed per investigator judgment and are subject to Agency review).
5. Audit follow-up is disruptive because minor items that are already corrected are reported to corporate management out of context.

There will always be a certain amount of tension between auditors and those whom they are auditing; however, corporate executives who rely on the audit services need to assure there are "partnerships" between managers of corporate audit programs and business unit managers. Roles need to be clearly defined and understood so that corporate interests are served. Audit findings need to be supported by facts and the auditees must be given the opportunity to respond to any deficiencies observed. Operational managers and their staffs should have a good understanding of the rules and policies that govern their operations and, generally, superior technical knowledge to that of the auditor. The auditors bring different perspective or "outside eyes" to an operation and should be expected to probe systems and question whether they are functioning as designed.

A. Internal Audit Communications

Long-standing FDA policy is that companies should have the opportunity to maintain internal audit programs that ferret out problems and assure their correction without interference from the Agency. Accordingly, FDA investigators have been advised to only request internal audit reports when investigating a serious health problem or upon the order of a court. It is therefore appropriate for companies to deny audit reports should an investigator request them. On the other hand, it makes a very positive statement to show an investigator a copy of the audit program and the schedule even though internal audits are not required by the drug CGMP rules.

Recently, a company had a consultant perform an internal audit and requested that the audit report be sent to its outside counsel because it would be protected under attorney–client privilege. This somewhat unusual report routing was due in part to a court ruling last year [Grand Jury Proceedings, 861 F. Supp. 386 (D. Md. 1994)] that both company and consultant internal audit reports had to be disclosed in response to a grand jury subpoena. The grand jury was investigating an FDA referral and violations of the Food, Drug and Cosmetic Act were involved. The case involved the possibility that false information had been submitted and that FDA inspections had been obstructed. Had the matter not involved obstruction of justice, the court probably would have declined to order the records produced in view of the FDA's policy not to ordinarily seek such records.

Several articles have been published about the above-mentioned case, and some suggested that attorneys participate in the review of all internal audit reports to ensure that such reports can be kept confidential under attorney–client privilege. One article suggested that the decision in the investigative Grand Jury situation could be extended to other types of government investigations. Of course, that is true, but does it mean companies have to have their lawyers review all quality assurance program functions and decisions? Such legal maneuvering should be unnecessary for companies that are acting in good faith to maintain strong quality assurance programs and to comply with the law. An internal audit program that uncovers manufacturing and QC deficiencies and tracks corrective actions demonstrates good faith, and the Food, Drug and Cosmetic Act, under Section 303(c) (4), exempts from criminal prosecution those who act in good faith. Communications about audit findings between corporate auditors and operational manages should not become any more constrained than they already are at many firms.

Probably the most important single issue to consider in evaluating a corporate program is: How should executive management be informed of audit activities? This is a touchy subject because audit programs require the support of executive management to be effective. The managers must be given enough information to evaluate the program and understand its merits; however, the audit program will be jeopardized if executive managers feel they must intervene when they hear of specific problems.

Executive managers should be regularly provided summary information, including: (1) the number of audits performed (with a listing of sites visited as an option); (2) whether the audit schedule is being conducted as planned; and (3) any corporate-wide problems and positive or negative trends.

It would be acceptable for such reports to also include positive audit findings or positive comments as to a site's responsiveness to an audit. On the other hand, specific adverse findings that are being corrected generally should not be reported. The frequency of such reports will vary depending on corporate management wishes, but should be at least quarterly for most firms. Should the manager of the audit group believe a situation represents potential legal problems, he or she should work with the division to schedule a meeting with executive management and counsel.

Routine internal audit reports should be provided to the management of the site audited and assistance provided, if necessary, for the sites to develop corrective action plans. Should there be an irresolvable disagreement between a division and the corporate audit group, the manager of the operating division, not the audit group, should raise the issue to corporate management. Audit groups need to be kept informed of all decisions relating to their findings to effectively monitor corrective actions. An audit group would report a specific issue to executive management only if they believe an uncorrected finding presents a potential liability for the company and the division has inappropriately represented the matter to management. In such an instance, the division would be informed in advance of the audit group's decision to make a report.

B. Cost Effectiveness of Audits

Looking at the very practical side of audits, we must ask ourselves whether internal audits make a difference. As is true with most quality assurance elements, it is most difficult to measure preventative activities in terms of the bottom line. Accordingly, companies that have good compliance records and few, if any, regulatory problems, frequently consider scaling back their quality systems, including audit programs. Perhaps the reason a Park case [*United States v. Park*, 421 U.S. 658 (1975)] is brought from time to time is because businesses become too preoccupied with the bottom line. Many companies that have trouble with approvals and face enforcement actions have badly flawed audit programs or no program at all. The rehabilitation programs that some firms have engaged in to achieve compliance appear more costly than maintaining a quality system that includes an effective internal audit component.

The primary objective of an audit program must be broadly understood by all parties as a system of working together to identify areas for improvement (rather than finding fault or engaging in autocratic criticism). Corporate auditors should be viewed as staff available to help line managers to do their jobs better. The audit group should be an extension of executive management leadership and not in any way diminish the responsibility and authority of division managers.

V. ROLE OF THE QUALITY ASSURANCE UNIT

A. Management—Separation of Quality Function

The Kefauver Harris Drug Amendments in 1962 provided the FDA with explicit authority [21 USC 351(a)(2)(B)] to promulgate drug GMP regulations. The first regulations under that section required a QC unit separate from production units. The preamble to the CGMPs for Finished Pharmaceuticals published in the Federal Register 9-29-78 provides the most recent interpretation, stating "The Commissioner intends to make the quality control unit responsible for ensuring that controls are implemented during manufacturing operations which assure drug product quality, not that the quality control unit actually perform each one of the duties." Elsewhere in the rule it says that neither the name of the unit nor its organizational structure is distinguished by the regulation. These comments suggest that the FDA agrees that businesses should develop quality programs that function well in view of their business requirements. Some organizational structures are no doubt more effective than others; however, there are so many variables, each firm may apply proven management concepts to their own needs, provided an independent quality unit provides the oversight required by the regulations.

B. Responsibility

In a one-person or family company, quality decisions can be based more on moral considerations than a managed decision process. However, even a one-person operation should adhere to the policy that, irrespective of any other duties, product quality must be assured. As companies grow to include hundreds or thousands of employees, quality management should periodically be re-evaluated and sometimes redirected.

Corporate management possesses the authority to establish quality standards that will assure competitiveness and to adjust resources as appropriate to meet those standards. It is public knowledge that the restructuring that went on at General Motors a few years ago resulted from products that were of such poor quality that they could not compete. During the same time period, the FDA insisted that a major pharmaceutical company enter into a Consent Decree of Permanent Injunction because a few of their divisions strayed significantly out of control. A number of that company's divisions were in substantial compliance with CGMPs; however, they also were impacted by the terms of the injunction. In such a situation, regulators are often reluctant to relieve a company from a civil or administrative action until they have corrected even minor deficiencies. In effect, that means a higher standard comes into play than the one that would be used to evaluate a firm during a routine inspection.

The FDA pre-approval inspection program can have an effect similar to that of an injunction in that a new product may be withheld from the market indefinitely pending corrections to FDA satisfaction. Top management of some companies ignore quality issues until after they are notified that approval will be withheld because of CGMP deficiencies. Common problems with such firms are that their written procedures are not understood or followed, validation is weak, and internal audit programs are ineffective.

Since the generic drug scandal, the FDA has had a special prosecutions task force assigned to the U.S. Attorney's Office in Baltimore, MD. There have been case referrals for grand jury investigation of several *Fortune 500* companies. Some now suggest that with a change in the political environment, the FDA will become less aggressive. That may be true, but it is also good reason for a major corporation to increase its own vigilance. It takes years for an effective quality system to decay through inattention; however, when one fails, the consequences can be disastrous.

At this point we might look at the Supreme Court's Park decision [*United States v. Park*, 421 U.S. 658 (1975)] for insight as to ultimate responsibility. In this case, the president of the corporation was charged with causing food to be held under unsanitary conditions in a warehouse. The president was not a participant in the wrongful act; indeed, he had management responsibility for 36,000 employees, 874 retail outlets, and 16 warehouses. However, the court found that "persons responsible for exercising supervisory authority have a duty not only to seek out and remedy violations but to prevent them, thus imposing upon that person a duty to take affirmative action."

A strong quality policy should be articulated by the CEO to demonstrate a commitment to affirmative action. A subordinate to the CEO should be delegated the responsibility for quality decisions, provided adequate resources to implement an effective program, and assured prompt access to the CEO in the event a critical quality problem needs to be discussed. The title of this person is unimportant as long as functional statements, procedures, and messages to all employees make the responsibility very clear. These concepts are widely accepted and have been discussed in preambles to the FDA GMP and GLP regulations and in the ISO 9000 quality standards and guidances.

Care must be taken to avoid any conflict of interest between quality management and staff and other business functions such as production and marketing. The FDA expects this to be documented as company policy. At the same time, it should be clear that quality personnel will not perform line functions. They are there to review, evaluate, verify, oversee, check, audit, or test equipment, systems, products, personnel, etc., and then, if necessary, to monitor change controls, corrective actions, and improvement plans. They may provide quality assurance advice or define problems to assist other units; however, they should not be expected to have greater technical expertise or to interfere in other than quality matters.

Over the past 10 years, "empowerment" may have been applied inappropriately at some regulated businesses through overdelegation of responsibility. Certainly, employees should be equipped, trained, and supported to conduct their responsibilities effectively; however, one of those responsibilities is to work within a system of checks and balances and support quality program objectives. Quality oversight and final product quality decisions, particularly in areas where the regulations are clear, must not be delegated to anyone other than quality personnel.

C. The Quality Organization

Depending on how a company's quality policy is stated, the scope of the quality assurance program can be limited to the production of products and services or it can extend to every employee and unit (including departments such as accounting). Even programs limited to products are not easy to organize. One must consider the size and location of operating units and the various kinds of products, processes, and technologies involved. Customer expectations, materials specifications, and laws and regulations may also impact the number of personnel needed and the way quality functions are subdivided into manageable work units. Sometimes the strengths and weaknesses of current managers and staff should be considered when deciding how to organize.

In larger firms, there is frequently overlap among quality and other support departments such as engineering, technical service, regulatory compliance, regulatory affairs, QC laboratory, and product development. Such interdepartmental functions must be clarified in procedures. In smaller and midsize firms, all of the separate departments may be units that are managed by a Vice President for Quality Assurance, or for Quality Assurance and Regulatory Affairs, or for Technical Services, or for Scientific Affairs, etc.

There are basic functions in most quality assurance departments. Control laboratories responsible for chemical, microbiological, and environmental testing are nearly always located in a quality department as a single QC division with different managers for each type of laboratory. Generally, quality departments have separate divisions or staffs responsible for activities or groups of activities such as the following:

1. documenting controls, including clearance and issuance of production records, procedures, specifications, etc.
2. internal and vendor audits
3. sampling, examination, and approval of materials, including packaging and labeling (often administered by the laboratory component of the department)
4. Material Review Board representative
5. verifying yields and other critical production data through production record audits
6. finished product release
7. accompanying FDA investigators and external auditors
8. administering or contributing to CGMP, safety, or other required training programs
9. assuring the investigations of product failures, process deviations, laboratory out-of-specification (OOS) findings, and consumer complaints
10. monitoring approval and implementation of corrective action plans and change controls
11. on-site verification of the performance of critical production operations such as clearing labeling equipment and lines

12. review and approval of the product development records and documents transferring a product from development to commercial production
13. validation/qualification protocols and summary reports acceptance
14. annual CGMP review

The following functions are sometimes performed by engineering or technical service departments with or without quality department approval:

1. statistical process control and trend analyses
2. calibration of instruments and equipment, including out-of-specification follow-up
3. analysis of reports of extraordinary maintenance and preventative maintenance failures

Depending on the size of the business, the R&D function may have its own quality assurance staff. Sometimes the chemistry support for development is provided by the QC laboratory. There are many possibilities for organizing a business and avoiding a conflict of interest in quality decision making. The independence of quality units must be assured by top management.

D. Vendor Audit Programs

The knowledge base a particular company has about its incoming materials is variable; therefore, the vendor quality program will need to be tailored to the company. For example, companies that are sponsors of NDAs or premarket applications (PMAs) have more than likely worked directly with drug substance or critical component suppliers to, among other things, profile impurities, perform degradation studies, and assure process validation. An over-the-counter (OTC) drug manufacturer may, at the other extreme, simply purchase compendial grade materials from supply houses. Certain components, excipients, containers, and closures may be custom formulated or designed for a product, whereas others may simply be stock items or often noncompendial items such as sucrose or medical grade silicon. Depending on the product line, a vendor quality assurance program may be more or less sophisticated to meet a company's needs.

International CGMP rules for pharmaceuticals, medical devices, and other regulated products require manufacturers to assure through an appropriate program or activity that components meet specifications and quality requirements. The ISO 9001 and ISO 9002 Quality Standards require manufacturers to select vendors on the basis of their ability to meet purchase specifications. By ISO 9004 definition, this includes meeting regulatory requirements and safety standards.

The FDA's CGMP regulations 21 CFR 211.84(a) through (e) require a manufacturer to test and approve or reject components, drug product containers, and closures. 21 CFR 211.84(d)(2) requires the manufacturer to test each component for conformity with written specifications for purity, strength, and quality or accept the supplier's report of analysis. 21 CFR 211.84(d)(3) requires the manufacturer to test containers and closures for conformance with all appropriate written procedures or accept the supplier's report of analysis. However, restrictions apply to accepting reports of analysis.

The restrictive conditions specified in the CGMP regulations for acceptance of a vendor's report of analysis for components: the manufacturer must (1) conduct at least one specific identity test on each lot received; and (2) establish the reliability of the suppliers through validation of supplier's test results at appropriate intervals. For containers and closures, a visual examination must be made on lots received and reliability established as above.

Originally, as documented in the preamble to the 1978 CGMP revision, the FDA expected a manufacturer to establish, through its own tests, that supplier reports of analyses on components were reliable. The manufacturer's and the supplier's results were expected to agree within specified limits over a period of time. Once the reliability of a supplier's data was established, the level of the manufacturer's validation testing could be reduced with an increased reliance on the supplier's reports. The preamble also said that manufacturers should have a system in place to assure continued reliability. The FDA currently has no written policy that addresses vendor certification beyond CGMP regulations; however, in recent years the Agency has taken the position that a process must be validated (among other reasons) to assure homogeneity of product when acceptance is based on testing of samples. As a practical matter, an audit may be a more cost-effective way of "validating" a vendor than the testing of many samples.

All pharmaceutical components should be included in a vendor quality assurance procedure or certification program before accepting (in lieu of testing incoming materials) vendors' certificates of analysis or inspection. This includes both drug substances and excipients, as well as containers and closures. The type and extent of evaluation before certifying acceptance should be dependent on the criticality of the material, previously demonstrated capability of the vendor, and conclusions reached during the certification process. While certification cannot be achieved without the cooperation and assistance of vendors, it should be made clear to all suppliers that the decision to certify, or to accept a third-party certification, is solely that of the purchaser. All or part of the following may be included in a program to assure that vendors' materials are of acceptable quality and that their certificates may be relied on: (1) vendor document review; (2) test methods verification; (3) on-site CGMP audit; (4) corrective action/consultation; and (5) notification of acceptance (or certification) of supplier.

E. Vendor Document Review

At minimum, there should be an evaluation of a vendor's marketing history for a material; a review of the source manufacturer's general organizational chart, quality manual, or SOP index; and pertinent regulatory records such as FDA-483s. For critical materials such as bulk active drug substances, document review should extend to product-specific flow charts, validation protocols and reports, summaries of conformance to test specifications, QC and quality assurance systems, and significant procedures such as those for change control and failure investigations.

When a manufacturer has referenced a vendor master file in a submission—or has collaborated with a vendor in submission of chemistry, manufacturing, and control data to FDA—the vendor should be requested to verify that updates have been submitted to the sponsor or FDA as required.

Quality Assurance should evaluate the documents and the vendor response. A visit to the vendor facility may be necessary should there be a language/translation problem or if for other reasons the documentation is not clear.

F. Test Methods Verification

Product specifications, standards, required equipment, and test methods must be evaluated to assure the capability exists, internally or by a contract laboratory, for QC to monitor or repeat the tests performed on a material by the source manufacturer. Generally, when a material is purported to comply with compendium specifications or when a basic testing or inspection procedure is used, the identification and testing procedures can be applied using minimal comparative testing. Samples of the vendor's material and copies of corresponding test results may be requested in the original letter or subsequent to the evaluation of documentation. If the vendor is a distributor, test results may have to be requested of the source manufacturer.

When sufficient data exist to assure that an incoming material has consistently conformed to specifications, the supplier may be certified or approved and scheduled for recertification at the appropriate interval.

G. On-Site GMP Audits

Audits are more productive when the auditor has had the opportunity to review in advance the type of documentation previously referred to. When vendor certification or approval is time sensitive, a qualified CGMP auditor may perform the audit by reviewing the conformance of quality assurance systems to CGMP regulations and applicable guidance documents made available by the FDA. A narrative report should be submitted for active drug substance vendor certification. When a source manufacturer of materials other than active drug substances has had the manufacturing site registered as conforming to ISO 9001 or ISO 9002, the registration may be useful. In deciding whether to accept an ISO registration, it is important to consider whether the material requires rigorous or general controls and whether the ISO audit team included someone familiar with the FDA regulatory requirements for the product class.

H. Use and Control of Contractors

Most pharmaceutical manufacturers now use contractors in the production and release of their products. Contractors provide services that the manufacturer would find prohibitively expensive or difficult to perform in-house. Industry pressures have driven many manufacturers to contract out certain laboratory tests, packaging and labeling operations, and sometimes the entire production. Contract Research Organizations (CROs) have become a major industry in the clinical testing of new drugs because, under the law, the firm that owns the drug product, such as the application holder, remains responsible for the product in the marketplace.

The relationship between the contractor and the pharmaceutical manufacturer is best when it approaches a partner-style relationship. In a true partnership, both parties contribute ideas and advice as to how the relationship can best work. The contractor has the expertise in the area of service provided. The manufacturer has the need to assure all procedures, tests, and controls are performed adequately and in compliance with all applicable regulations.

Drug products must always meet FDA and other regulatory standards. These standards include all commitments made in an application, IND, or DMF, as well as general requirements such as the CGMPs. The holder of the application (applicant) is primarily responsible for the product irrespective of any contract agreements. Simply put, if there is a problem regarding the product, including adulteration or misbranding, it is the applicant who will be contacted by the FDA and required to provide information regarding the product, its components, and the manufacturing process.

The contractor performing a manufacturing step is responsible for the work performed. In the event of a product adulteration, the FDA will hold the firm where the deviation(s) occurred responsible for violations of the CGMP regulations (21 CFR 210 and 211) that pertain to those services. However, the contractor and the application holder will be held jointly responsible for processes performed by the contractor to the extent that each party contributed to the violations. Performance of each party will be considered in determining whether one or both parties are subject to regulatory action for failure to comply with CGMPs (reference AAC # for Compliance Policy Guide 7150.16).

It is in the best interest of the applicant to perform due diligence in the selection of any contractor, as well as to audit the contractors to ensure they meet the regulatory requirements and the contractual commitments. Written agreements should include not only a detailed description of what will be provided by the contract manufacturers (e.g., manufacturing and testing), they should also include how the commitments to the application and the FDA regulations will be achieved.

For manufacturing, details such as how the applicant controls the production procedures—including shipment and receipt of components, the use of specific SOPs controlling all aspects of the process, authorities for release of components, in-process materials, and final product—should be covered in the contract. The contract should also cover the components (active and inactive substances); specifications (and who has the authority to set specifications); how and by whom sampling is performed; components testing and acceptance criteria; vendor certification/audits; laboratory test procedures; and approval authorities. Validation issues, such as who is responsible for performing and approving validation and cleaning validation protocols and studies, should also be addressed.

There must also be a specified change control procedure. No changes should be made without adequate modification, deliberation, and written approvals. To correct inadvertent shifts in performance capability, there should be periodic contract reviews and audits of the operation or services covered by the contract.

In the service contract area, providers are often expected to perform functions that have not been specified. CROs, for example, may contract to distribute the study drug, verify case reports, and ensure that informed consent is documented.

However, accounting for unused study drug and monitoring Institutional Review Board (IRB) activities may not be part of the contract. This has led to firms finding that these issues remain ignored until the end of a study, when it is difficult or not possible to reconstruct events. Similarly, contractors calibrating instruments may be able to readjust out of specification instruments but are not in a position to investigate the products that may have been adversely affected by the use of defective equipment.

It is incumbent on the pharmaceutical manufacturer to ensure that the use of outside contractors is well defined in their own procedures and the contract. It is also important that the manufacturer audit, check, and verify that the contractor is performing according to the contract and all applicable standards. The manufacturer should also carefully review their own internal procedures to ensure that timely and adequate follow-up is made to findings and actions of the contractor.

I. Corrective Action/Consultation

Any corrective actions that need to be accomplished before further consideration should be documented and agreed upon. Time frames should be established for all necessary actions, including any overall quality system, test method verification, or CGMP issues that need to be resolved by the vendor. Communications channels with vendor representatives should be documented to integrate change control, quality management, and quality improvement between supplier and customer.

J. Notification

When requirements are reviewed and agreed upon, the vendor may be notified of the determination of acceptability and/or orders may be placed. Some companies issue a certificate that the vendor has demonstrated the capability to produce to the mutually agreed upon requirements and effected procedures that will be used to forward the agreed-upon change reports, reports of analysis, or other records. If a prospective vendor is found to be unacceptable because a quality system is found to be inadequate, the company should be informed by letter.

A program could be structured to perform all of these steps in sequence and document step-by-step decisions on a form. Such decisions may include omitting a subsequent step or intensifying coverage of an area of concern. Form entries for each step may document whether the vendor was found acceptable, conditionally acceptable, or unacceptable. The resolution of conditional acceptances may be attended to by review of corrective actions and appropriate documentation.

Depending on whether the desired procedure is a "certification" program or an internal vendor acceptance procedure, notification may consist of issuing a certificate or simply authorizing (under a written procedure) the purchasing department to place an order. Simultaneous or interactive evaluations of quality documents, audits, and records may be made when a material is urgently needed; however, final approval of a vendor should not take place until all decisions have been documented and approved by the Quality Assurance department.

A recertification or vendor quality schedule review may be specified for each type of material. Recertification may be based on review of communications with suppliers about process or methods changes, review of inspection/test history for the material, on-site audit, third-party audit certification, or a combination of these activities. An initial certification or vendor acceptance should require a more comprehensive evaluation than when a purchaser has experience with a supplier.

K. Resource Commitment

Because CGMPs require firms to follow their own written procedures, it would be unwise to create vendor quality assurance program procedures without ensuring that resources will be available for implementing and accomplishing them. Likewise, recertification must take resources into consideration, but for the long term.

VI. THE FINAL CHECK

With all of the above in mind, the firm must decide before the pre-approval inspection just how to go about conducting a "last check" to ensure that everything is in place and that they are prepared. Many firms use a variety of approaches, including: (1) the use of outside consultants to conduct a CGMP internal audit; (2) the use of outside consultants to conduct an application audit; and (3) the use of internal teams to do both an internal audit and application audit.

The key is to do a final reality check on the firm's readiness just before the FDA's arrival. The person(s) conducting this final check must be competent in the areas being audited and must have the confidence and support of firm management. Findings must be quickly acted upon by the firm.

REFERENCES

1. 21 CFR—Parts 210 and 211 Regulations, Current Good Manufacturing Practice in Manufacturing, Processing, Packing or Holding of Drugs; General, and Current Good Manufacturing Practices for Finished Pharmaceuticals.
2. FDA, *Guideline on The Preparation of Investigational New Drug Products*, March 1991.
3. FDA, *FDA Compliance Program Guidance Manual-Compliance Program— 7346.832—Pre-Approval Inspections/Investigations*, published annually.
4. Federal Food Drug and Cosmetic Act as amended 1998.
5. FDA, *FDA Guide to Inspections of Pharmaceutical Quality Control Laboratories*, July 1993.
6. FDA, *FDA Guide to Inspection of Dosage Form Drug Manufacturers—CGMP's*, October 1993.
7. FDA, *Guide to Inspections of Oral Solid Dosage Forms Pre/Post Approval Issues for Development and Validation*, January 1994.
8. FDA, *FDA Guide to Inspections of Bulk Pharmaceutical Chemicals*, September 1991.
9. Leonard Steinborn, *GMP/ISO 9000 Quality Audit Manual*, Interpharm Press, Buffalo Grove, IL.

Index